Polyvagal-Informed Trauma Therapy

A Comprehensive Guide to Nervous System
Assessment, Co-Regulation, and Integration with
Evidence-Based Modalities

Doreen Anna Richmond

Table of Contents

Table of Contents

Chapter 1: The Polyvagal Framework

Your body knows things your mind hasn't figured out yet. Right now, as you sit reading this, your nervous system is running millions of calculations, deciding if you're safe enough to focus on these words or if you need to scan for danger. This happens completely outside your awareness, faster than thought, through an ancient system that's kept mammals alive for millions of years.

The Polyvagal Theory, developed by Stephen Porges in the mid-1990s, gives us a revolutionary way to understand this system. It's not just another theory to add to your clinical toolkit—it's a fundamental shift in how we understand human behavior, trauma, and the healing process. For therapists, this framework explains why talking about feelings doesn't always help, why some clients can't make eye contact, and why the quality of your presence matters more than your techniques.

What makes this theory so powerful is that it bridges biology and psychology in a way that makes immediate clinical sense. When you understand that your client's symptoms are actually their nervous system's adaptive responses to threat, everything changes. You stop seeing resistance and start seeing protection. You stop pushing for change and start creating safety. You stop treating symptoms and start working with the wisdom of the body.

Evolution and Neurophysiology of the Autonomic Nervous System

Let's start with a story that goes back 500 million years. Long before humans walked the earth, before dinosaurs roamed, the earliest vertebrates faced a fundamental challenge: how to survive in a dangerous world. Their solution was elegant—when faced with

1

overwhelming threat, shut everything down. Conserve energy. Play dead. Wait it out.

This ancient survival strategy, mediated by what we now call the dorsal vagal complex, is still with us today. It's the unmyelinated portion of the vagus nerve that originates in the dorsal motor nucleus. When activated, it dramatically reduces metabolic demands—heart rate plummets, breathing slows, digestion stops. In fish and reptiles, this is adaptive. A turtle pulls into its shell. A lizard freezes perfectly still. For these creatures, immobilization equals survival.

Fast forward a few hundred million years to the age of early mammals. These warm-blooded creatures needed more options than just freezing. They developed what we call the sympathetic nervous system—the ability to mobilize, to take action. This system floods the body with stress hormones, speeds up the heart, dilates the pupils, and sends blood rushing to the large muscles. Now, when threatened, mammals could fight back or run away. Action became a survival strategy.

But here's where it gets really interesting. About 200 million years ago, mammals developed something revolutionary—a myelinated branch of the vagus nerve originating in the nucleus ambiguus. This "smart vagus" did something no other nervous system could do: it linked cardiac regulation with the muscles of social communication. The same neural pathways that calm your heart also control your ability to make eye contact, modulate your voice, and orient your head to listen.

Think about what this means. Evolution found a way to use connection as a survival strategy. A baby's cry brings the caregiver. A soothing voice calms a frightened child. A reassuring face tells us we're safe. This social engagement system, unique to mammals, allows us to co-regulate with others—to literally use another nervous system to help regulate our own.

The genius of Porges' theory is recognizing that we didn't lose these older systems as we evolved. Instead, we built new systems on top of old ones. All three systems—the ancient dorsal vagal, the sympathetic, and the newer ventral vagal—are active in your body right now. They work in a hierarchy, with newer systems inhibiting older ones when we feel safe, but older systems taking over when we detect threat.

This evolutionary perspective completely reframes how we understand trauma responses. When someone dissociates during a flashback, they're not weak or broken—their nervous system is using an ancient survival strategy. When someone can't stop scanning for danger, they're not choosing to be hypervigilant—their sympathetic system is doing what it evolved to do. And when someone struggles to connect after trauma, it's because their social engagement system has gone offline in service of survival.

The Three Neural Circuits: Ventral Vagal, Sympathetic, and Dorsal Vagal Pathways

Now we get to the heart of what makes Polyvagal Theory so clinically useful—understanding the three distinct states our nervous system can inhabit. Each state isn't just a different level of arousal; it's a completely different way of being in the world, with its own perceptions, behaviors, and possibilities for connection.

The Ventral Vagal State is our home base when we feel safe. This is the state of social engagement, where all our mammalian superpowers come online. In this state, your heart rate variability is high—not a racing heart, but a flexible, responsive heart that speeds up and slows down with your breathing. Your middle ear muscles are tuned to human voice frequencies. Your face is mobile and expressive. You can make eye contact without it feeling threatening or overwhelming.

But it's more than just physiology. In ventral vagal, your whole experience of the world changes. Colors seem brighter. Time moves at a normal pace. You can think about the future without panic and the past without getting stuck. You have access to what we might call executive function—the ability to plan, prioritize, and make

3

decisions. Creativity flows. Play becomes possible. You can be intimate without fear.

In therapy, clients in ventral vagal are a joy to work with. They can tolerate difficult emotions without being overwhelmed. They can reflect on their experiences with curiosity rather than judgment. They make connections between past and present. They can receive support and offer it in return. This is where healing happens—not through force or will, but through the natural repair processes that come online when we feel safe.

The Sympathetic State is all about mobilization. This is your body's action system, designed to help you escape or overcome threat. Within milliseconds of detecting danger—and remember, this detection happens below conscious awareness—your entire physiology reorganizes for action. Your heart rate jumps. Blood pressure rises. Pupils dilate to take in more information. Blood flows away from your digestive system and toward your large muscles. Stress hormones flood your system.

In this state, your perception narrows. You literally see less peripherally as your vision tunnels toward the threat. Your hearing changes too—you become more sensitive to low-frequency sounds (predator sounds) and less able to hear human voice frequencies. Time seems to speed up or slow down. Everything becomes about the threat—finding it, facing it, or fleeing from it.

Clients in sympathetic activation are restless, agitated, unable to settle. They might pace your office or fidget constantly. Their thoughts race. They interrupt, talk over you, or can't seem to hear what you're saying. Some describe feeling "wired but tired"—exhausted but unable to rest. Others report a constant sense of impending doom, like something terrible is about to happen even though they can't say what.

Here's what's crucial to understand: sympathetic activation isn't pathology. It's an adaptive response that has saved countless lives throughout evolution. The problem isn't the response itself—it's when

4

we get stuck there. When the nervous system can't find its way back to safety after the threat has passed. When mobilization becomes a chronic state rather than a temporary response.

The Dorsal Vagal State takes us into the realm of immobilization. This is our most ancient defense, the one we share with reptiles and fish. When we can't fight, can't flee, and can't connect our way to safety, this old system takes over. It's the ultimate conservation mode—shutting down everything non-essential to preserve energy and wait out the threat.

In dorsal vagal, heart rate and blood pressure drop dramatically. Digestion slows or stops. You might feel nauseous or have digestive problems. Your body feels heavy, like you're moving through molasses. Breathing becomes shallow. You might feel cold, especially in your extremities. Some people describe it as feeling like they're wrapped in cotton wool or behind a glass wall.

But the subjective experience is even more profound. In dorsal vagal shutdown, you disconnect—from your body, from others, from yourself. Emotions flatten. Nothing seems to matter. You might watch yourself from outside your body or feel like you're not really present. Some clients describe it as "going away" or "checking out." Others say they feel nothing—not sad, not scared, just... nothing.

This state serves an important survival function. If you can't escape a predator, playing dead might save your life. In situations of inescapable trauma—childhood abuse, captivity, severe accidents— dorsal shutdown can be protective, taking us out of an unbearable experience. But like sympathetic activation, problems arise when we get stuck here, when shutdown becomes our default rather than a last resort.

Neuroception: The Unconscious Detection of Safety and Danger

Here's where Polyvagal Theory gets really fascinating. Your nervous system is constantly scanning your environment, inside and out, evaluating whether you're safe or in danger. Porges calls this process "neuroception," and it happens completely outside your conscious awareness, processed through ancient brain structures that don't have direct connections to the thinking parts of your brain.

Neuroception works through multiple channels simultaneously. It's monitoring your internal state—are you hungry, tired, in pain? It's scanning your environment—what's the lighting like, are there escape routes, are there sudden movements or loud noises? And crucially, it's reading other nervous systems—is that person's face friendly or threatening, is their voice melodic or harsh, is their body posture open or closed?

This scanning happens through subcortical pathways, particularly structures like the periaqueductal gray and the superior colliculus. These ancient brain regions process information and trigger responses faster than your cortex can form a thought. By the time you consciously register that something feels "off," your body has already started responding—shifting your autonomic state, preparing for action or shutdown.

For trauma survivors, neuroception often becomes miscalibrated. The nervous system, shaped by experiences of threat, starts detecting danger everywhere. A door slamming becomes a sign of violence. A neutral face looks angry. A friendly touch feels threatening. The system that evolved to keep us safe becomes hypervigilant, constantly triggering defensive responses to non-threatening stimuli.

Consider James, a combat veteran. He knows intellectually that the grocery store is safe, but his neuroception disagrees. The fluorescent lights remind his nervous system of the harsh lighting in combat zones. The unpredictable movements of other shoppers trigger surveillance responses. The feeling of being boxed in by aisles activates escape planning. His thinking brain says "safe," but his nervous system screams "danger," and guess which one controls his physiological response?

This mismatch between cognitive understanding and neuroceptive evaluation creates profound suffering. Clients will say, "I know I'm safe, but I can't feel safe." They're describing the conflict between their cortical processing and their subcortical threat detection. And here's the thing—you can't think your way out of neuroception. You can't logic your nervous system into feeling safe.

What you can do is provide the nervous system with explicit cues of safety. This is where the therapeutic environment becomes crucial. Soft lighting instead of harsh fluorescents. Comfortable seating with clear sight lines to the door. A therapist who speaks with prosody, makes appropriate eye contact, and whose own regulated nervous system broadcasts safety. These environmental and relational factors speak directly to neuroception, bypassing the need for cognitive processing.

The Social Engagement System and Its Role in Healing

The social engagement system is perhaps Porges' most revolutionary contribution to our understanding of human behavior. This system, unique to mammals, integrates the neural regulation of the heart with the neural regulation of the muscles of the face and head. It's what allows us to use social connection as a biological strategy for calming our nervous system.

The anatomy is fascinating. The myelinated vagus nerve, originating in the nucleus ambiguus, doesn't work alone. It's functionally linked with cranial nerves that control facial expression, vocalization, listening, and head turning. When this integrated system is online, we can engage in the nuanced social communication that defines mammalian, and especially human, interaction.

Think about what happens when you're comforting a distressed friend. Without conscious thought, your face softens. Your voice takes on a particular quality—lower in pitch, with more melodic variation. You orient your body toward them, maybe tilting your head slightly. Your own breathing slows and deepens. All of these changes happen automatically, orchestrated by your social engagement system.

But here's the magic—these changes in you trigger changes in your friend. Their nervous system, through neuroception, detects your cues of safety. Their heart rate starts to slow. Their breathing deepens. The muscles of their face begin to soften. Without a word being spoken, your regulated nervous system has begun to regulate theirs. This is co-regulation, and it's fundamental to how we heal from trauma.

The social engagement system explains why the therapeutic relationship is so much more than just rapport. When a therapist maintains their own ventral vagal state—staying genuinely present, regulated, and engaged—they offer their nervous system as a co-regulatory resource. The client's nervous system, starved for safety, can begin to borrow the therapist's regulation, using it as a bridge back to their own social engagement capacity.

But trauma often damages the social engagement system. Early relational trauma, in particular, can compromise our ability to accurately read social cues, to produce appropriate facial expressions, or to modulate our voice effectively. These aren't just social skill deficits—they're neurobiological injuries to the very system we need for connection and co-regulation.

This is why many trauma survivors struggle with relationships. It's not that they don't want connection—in fact, the need for safe connection is a biological imperative. It's that their social engagement system has been compromised, making connection feel dangerous or impossible. They might avoid eye contact because it triggers threat responses. Their voice might be flat because prosody requires ventral vagal activation. They might misread friendly faces as threatening because their neuroception is tuned for danger.

Clinical Implications for Trauma Treatment

So what does all this mean for how we actually work with clients? Polyvagal Theory doesn't just give us a new way to understand trauma—it fundamentally changes how we approach treatment. Instead of seeing symptoms as problems to eliminate, we understand

8

them as adaptive responses that once served survival. Instead of pushing for change, we focus first on creating safety.

Assessment through a Polyvagal lens means paying attention to autonomic states, not just symptoms. Where does this client spend most of their time—in hypervigilant sympathetic activation, in collapsed dorsal vagal shutdown, or do they have access to ventral vagal regulation? Can they move flexibly between states based on actual environmental demands, or are they stuck in defensive responses?

You can assess this through observation. Notice their breathing—is it shallow and rapid (sympathetic) or barely there (dorsal)? What about eye contact—is it intense and scanning (sympathetic), avoidant (dorsal), or warm and flexible (ventral)? Listen to their voice—is it pressured and loud, flat and monotonous, or does it have melody and variation? These observations tell you more about their nervous system state than any standardized assessment.

Treatment sequencing becomes crucial. If someone is stuck in dorsal shutdown, you can't just jump into trauma processing. Their nervous system literally doesn't have the resources online for integration. You need to first help them back into their window of tolerance, perhaps through gentle activation—movement, temperature, rhythm. Only when they have access to ventral vagal regulation can you begin to work with traumatic material.

The therapeutic relationship isn't just important—it's the primary intervention. Your regulated nervous system, your genuine presence, your attuned responses—these provide the co-regulatory experiences that help repair the client's capacity for connection. This isn't about being nice or warm. It's about offering your social engagement system as a neurobiological resource for healing.

This means your own regulation matters enormously. If you're in sympathetic activation—rushed, stressed, overwhelmed—your client's neuroception will detect those cues of danger. If you're in dorsal shutdown—going through the motions, checked out, disconnected—they'll sense that too. Your ventral vagal presence, your genuine regulated engagement, is one of the most powerful tools you have.

Bottom-up interventions become essential. While cognitive approaches can be helpful when someone has access to ventral vagal regulation, they're less effective when the nervous system is in a defensive state. Somatic approaches, breathing exercises, movement, rhythm, touch (when appropriate)—these work directly with the nervous system, bypassing the need for cortical processing. They speak the language of the body, the language of the autonomic nervous system.

Essential Concepts for Practice

Understanding Polyvagal Theory changes how you sit with clients. You start to see the wisdom in their symptoms rather than pathology. You recognize that resistance is often the nervous system protecting against overwhelm. You understand that progress isn't always linear because nervous systems shaped by trauma need time to learn that safety is possible.

This framework helps explain why some days clients can process difficult material while other days they can't access those resources. It's not resistance or regression—it's autonomic state. Their nervous system might be responding to cues of danger you're not even aware of—a change in barometric pressure, an anniversary date, a smell that triggered implicit memory.

Most importantly, Polyvagal Theory gives us a map for healing that honors the body's wisdom. Instead of trying to override defensive responses, we work with them. Instead of pushing through resistance, we respect it as protection. Instead of focusing solely on cognitive insight, we help the nervous system learn, through repeated experiences of safety, that connection is possible again.

The journey from trauma to healing is really a journey of reclaiming flexibility in our autonomic nervous system. It's about expanding the range of states we can inhabit and building our capacity to return to safety after activation. It's about reconnecting with our mammalian birthright—the ability to use connection with others to regulate our own nervous system. And it starts with understanding that every symptom, every defense, every seemingly maladaptive behavior is actually the nervous system's attempt to ensure survival.

Chapter 2: The Neurobiology of Trauma Through a Polyvagal Lens

Sarah sits across from me, describing her life with the kind of detached precision that immediately tells me her nervous system has checked out. "I do everything I'm supposed to do," she says, her voice flat as week-old soda. "Work, kids, bills, groceries. But it feels like I'm watching someone else's life through a window. Like I'm not really here." Her body is so still it's almost disturbing. No gestures, no shifts in position, barely any blinking. This isn't calm—this is collapse.

Traditional psychology might label Sarah with depression, dissociation, maybe PTSD. And sure, those labels have their place. But they don't capture what's actually happening in her body. Through a Polyvagal lens, I see something different: a nervous system that learned to survive unbearable experiences by shutting down the very circuits that make us feel alive. Her symptoms aren't the problem—they're her body's solution to a problem we haven't solved yet.

This is the radical shift Polyvagal Theory offers us. Instead of seeing pathology, we see adaptation. Instead of dysfunction, we see protection. Instead of resistance, we see a nervous system doing exactly what it evolved to do: prioritize survival over everything else, including feeling, connecting, and living fully. Once you understand this, everything about trauma treatment changes.

How PTSD Symptoms Reflect Autonomic Nervous System Dysregulation

PTSD isn't really a disorder—it's a nervous system that got stuck in survival mode and can't find its way back to safety. Every single symptom in the diagnostic criteria makes perfect sense when you understand it as an autonomic nervous system response that won't turn off.

Take hypervigilance. From a Polyvagal perspective, this is sympathetic nervous system activation that won't downregulate. The body is constantly scanning for danger, muscles ready to spring into action, stress hormones keeping everything on high alert. The person isn't choosing to be paranoid or anxious—their nervous system is stuck in a state that says "danger is imminent" even when their thinking brain knows they're safe.

Or consider emotional numbing, what the DSM calls "diminished interest or participation in activities." This isn't apathy or not caring— it's dorsal vagal shutdown. The nervous system has decided that feeling is too dangerous, that the only way to survive is to disconnect from emotions, from the body, from others. It's not a cognitive choice. It's a biological state.

Flashbacks? That's the nervous system detecting some cue—a smell, a sound, a sensation—that it associates with the original trauma. Neuroception picks up this cue and instantly shifts the entire system into the defensive response that was active during the trauma. The person isn't remembering the trauma; they're re-experiencing the physiological state of the trauma. Their body literally can't tell the difference between then and now.

Sleep disturbances make perfect sense too. How can you sleep deeply when your nervous system believes you're in danger? Sleep requires a certain level of ventral vagal activation—the state of safety and connection. If your nervous system is stuck in sympathetic arousal or dorsal shutdown, real restorative sleep becomes impossible. You might pass out from exhaustion, but that's not the same as sleep.

Even the avoidance symptoms are autonomic responses. When your nervous system has learned that certain places, people, or situations trigger overwhelming physiological responses, avoidance isn't a choice—it's survival. The body is saying, "That thing almost killed us once. We're not going near it again." This isn't conscious. It's programmed into the nervous system at a level way below thought.

What we call "negative alterations in cognitions and mood" are really descriptions of how different autonomic states shape our perception and meaning-making. In chronic dorsal vagal shutdown, the world literally looks different. Colors are muted. Time moves strangely. Nothing feels real or meaningful. It's not that the person is choosing negative thoughts—their nervous system state is creating a particular lens through which they experience reality.

Understanding Dissolution and Hierarchical Responses to Threat

Porges borrowed a concept from John Hughlings Jackson, a 19th-century neurologist, called "dissolution." Jackson observed that when the nervous system is under extreme stress, we lose our most recently evolved capacities first and fall back on older, more primitive responses. It's like evolution in reverse.

Here's how it works. Under normal circumstances, our ventral vagal system—our social engagement system—keeps the older defensive systems in check. We can stay calm, connected, and thoughtful even when facing challenges because this newer system inhibits the older fight-flight-freeze responses. But when we detect serious threat, this inhibition is released, and the older systems come online.

First, we lose social engagement. The muscles of the face become less mobile. The voice loses its melody. Eye contact becomes difficult. We can't really hear what others are saying because our middle ear muscles have shifted to detect predator sounds rather than human voice. We're still functional, but connection becomes almost impossible.

If the threat continues or escalates, we move into sympathetic mobilization. Now we're in full fight-or-flight mode. The thinking brain goes offline—this is why people make such poor decisions when they're activated. Everything becomes about the threat. Time perception changes. Pain sensitivity decreases (so we can keep fighting or running even if injured). Digestion stops. Immune function suppresses. The body is burning through resources at an unsustainable rate.

If we can't fight or flee our way to safety, the nervous system makes a last-ditch survival move: dorsal vagal shutdown. This is like pulling the emergency brake. Everything slows down dramatically. Heart rate and blood pressure drop. Breathing becomes shallow. We disconnect from our body, from our feelings, from the world around us. In extreme cases, people faint—the ultimate immobilization response.

Now here's what's crucial for understanding trauma: this dissolution can happen in response to perceived threat, not just actual threat. For someone with trauma, a trigger can initiate this entire cascade. Within seconds, they can go from feeling relatively okay to complete sympathetic overwhelm or dorsal collapse. They're not being dramatic or attention-seeking. Their nervous system is running an old program that once saved their life.

The hierarchy also explains why some interventions work sometimes and not others. If someone is in dorsal shutdown, you can't just talk to them about their feelings—the circuits needed for that kind of processing are offline. You need to first help them back into a state where those circuits are available. This is why body-based, bottom-up approaches are so important in trauma work.

The Vagus Nerve as a Bi-Directional Communication Pathway

Here's something that blows people's minds when they first learn it: 80% of the vagus nerve fibers are sensory, carrying information from the body up to the brain. Only 20% carry motor commands from the brain down to the body. This means your body is constantly telling your brain how to feel, not the other way around.

This bi-directional communication explains why body-based interventions can be so powerful for trauma. When you change your breathing pattern, you're not just moving air—you're sending signals up the vagus nerve that tell your brain whether you're safe or in danger. Slow, deep breathing with a longer exhale activates the ventral vagus, signaling safety. Rapid, shallow breathing activates sympathetic responses, signaling threat.

The same is true for posture. Stand in a collapsed, protective posture, and your body sends signals of defeat and shutdown up to your brain. Stand with an open chest and lifted head, and different signals travel up the vagus, potentially shifting you toward a more regulated state. This isn't about "power posing" or faking it—it's about understanding that the body is constantly informing the brain about our state.

This bi-directional pathway also explains why trauma gets "stuck" in the body. The body holds patterns of activation or shutdown that continuously signal danger to the brain, even when the threat is long past. A chronically tight diaphragm keeps sending "danger" signals. Collapsed shoulders keep signaling "defeat." These body patterns maintain the trauma response long after the traumatic event.

The gut-brain connection is part of this too. The vagus nerve extensively innervates our digestive system, and our gut contains more neurons than our spinal cord. When people say they have a "gut feeling" about something, they're describing real neural communication. Trauma often disrupts this communication, leading to digestive problems, food sensitivities, and the loss of those intuitive gut feelings that help us navigate the world.

Understanding this bi-directional communication changes how we approach treatment. Instead of trying to think our way out of trauma, we can work directly with the body to send new signals up to the brain. Breathing exercises, movement, touch, rhythm—these aren't just coping strategies. They're ways of directly communicating with the nervous system in its own language.

Fetal Patterns and Early Trauma: Developmental Considerations

The autonomic nervous system begins developing in utero, and the experiences of those nine months profoundly shape how it functions for the rest of our lives. The fetus is already practicing the detection

16

of safety and threat, already learning patterns of regulation or dysregulation based on the mother's state and the intrauterine environment.

When a pregnant mother experiences chronic stress, her elevated cortisol crosses the placenta and affects the developing nervous system of her baby. The fetus learns, at the deepest biological level, that the world is dangerous. Their nervous system develops with a bias toward detecting threat, with a lowered threshold for triggering defensive responses.

Research has shown that babies born to mothers who experienced trauma during pregnancy often show signs of autonomic dysregulation from birth. They might be difficult to soothe, have trouble with sleep, or show heightened startle responses. Their nervous systems are already primed for danger before they even take their first breath.

The birth process itself can be traumatic, especially when there are complications. Being stuck in the birth canal, experiencing oxygen deprivation, or being separated from mother immediately after birth—these experiences can trigger massive dorsal vagal responses in the newborn. The nervous system learns that helplessness and immobilization are paired with life threat, a pairing that can persist throughout life.

Early attachment relationships continue this developmental process. A baby's nervous system literally develops in relationship with their caregiver's nervous system. Through thousands of moments of co-regulation—or missed co-regulation—the infant learns whether connection is safe, whether their needs will be met, whether the world is predictable and manageable.

When caregivers are consistently available and attuned, the baby's nervous system learns to expect co-regulation. They develop a robust ventral vagal system and the capacity to recover from stress. But when caregivers are absent, dysregulated, or frightening, the baby's nervous system develops along different lines. They might become

17

hypervigilant, always watching for danger. Or they might collapse into shutdown, learning early that their needs won't be met.

These early patterns become the template for all future relationships. A nervous system that learned connection is dangerous will struggle with intimacy throughout life, not because of conscious beliefs but because of deep biological programming. This is why talk therapy alone often isn't enough for developmental trauma—we need to work at the level of the nervous system, creating new experiences of safe connection that can gradually rewire these early patterns.

Breaking the Shame Cycle Through Physiological Understanding

One of the most profound gifts of Polyvagal Theory is how it dissolves shame. When people understand that their responses to trauma are biological, not personal failures, something shifts. The story changes from "What's wrong with me?" to "My nervous system was trying to protect me."

Take the freeze response. So many trauma survivors carry devastating shame about not fighting back or not running away. They torture themselves with thoughts like "I should have done something" or "I just let it happen." But when they understand that freeze is an involuntary nervous system response—that their body made a split-second calculation that fighting or fleeing would be more dangerous—the shame begins to lift.

I've seen combat veterans sob with relief when they learn about dorsal vagal shutdown. Finally, they understand why they "froze" in combat situations. It wasn't cowardice. Their nervous system determined, based on the overwhelming threat, that immobilization was the best survival strategy. They didn't choose it any more than they chose for their heart to beat.

The same is true for people who responded to trauma with what looks like compliance or even participation. When you're in a state of dorsal vagal shutdown, you might appear calm or cooperative, but inside you're literally not there. You've dissociated as a survival strategy.

18

Understanding this biological reality can free people from years of self-blame about "going along with" their abuse.

Even symptoms that seem completely irrational make sense through this lens. The client who can't stop washing their hands isn't "crazy"— their nervous system is trying to create some sense of control in a world that feels dangerous. The person who can't leave their house isn't weak—their nervous system has decided that home is the only safe place and is protecting them from perceived threat.

This physiological understanding also helps with the shame of not being able to "just get over it." When you understand that trauma changes the nervous system at a biological level, you realize that healing isn't about willpower or positive thinking. It's about gradually creating new neural pathways, teaching the nervous system through repeated experiences that safety is possible.

The Path Forward

Understanding trauma through a Polyvagal lens fundamentally changes how we approach healing. We stop seeing symptoms as problems and start seeing them as solutions. We stop pushing for change and start creating conditions for change. We stop fighting the nervous system and start working with its inherent wisdom.

This perspective brings tremendous hope. If trauma responses are learned patterns in the nervous system, then new patterns can be learned. If the nervous system became dysregulated through overwhelming experiences, it can become regulated again through healing experiences. The same neuroplasticity that allowed trauma to shape the nervous system allows healing to reshape it.

But this healing doesn't happen through insight alone. It happens through experiences—experiences of safety, of connection, of successful mobilization, of coming back to calm. Each time someone moves from activation back to regulation, they're teaching their nervous system that it's possible to recover. Each moment of genuine connection is rewiring the social engagement system. Each time they stay present instead of dissociating, they're building new neural pathways.

The journey isn't linear. Nervous systems shaped by trauma are protective, and for good reason. They've learned that letting guard down is dangerous. So healing happens in spirals, with apparent setbacks that are actually the nervous system testing whether this new safety is real. Understanding this helps both clinicians and clients stay patient with the process.

Most importantly, this framework reminds us that healing happens in relationship. Our nervous systems were shaped in relationship—whether with caregivers, perpetrators, or the absence of connection—and they heal in relationship too. The therapeutic relationship becomes a laboratory for new experiences of safe connection, for learning that it's possible to be seen, to be vulnerable, to be human without being hurt.

Chapter 3: Creating Safety in the Therapeutic Environment

A colleague once asked me, "What's the most important thing in your therapy room?" Without hesitation, I answered, "The feeling of safety." Not the credentials on the wall, not the theoretical orientation, not even the specific interventions I use. Safety. Because without safety, nothing else matters. A dysregulated nervous system can't heal, can't learn, can't connect. It can only protect.

But here's what most therapists don't realize: safety isn't just about what we say or even how we say it. Safety is communicated through a thousand tiny details that our clients' nervous systems detect and evaluate before a single word is spoken. The height of your chair relative to theirs. The quality of light in the room. The distance between you. Whether they can see the door. These aren't just preferences—they're neurobiological needs that directly impact whether your client's nervous system decides you're safe enough to trust with their pain.

Through a Polyvagal lens, creating safety becomes a precise, intentional practice. We're not just being nice or creating a pleasant atmosphere. We're actively communicating to our clients' neuroception—that unconscious threat detection system—that this space, this relationship, this moment is safe enough for healing to begin.

Removing Cues of Danger in Clinical Settings

Your client's nervous system starts evaluating safety the moment they enter your building. Is the waiting room exposed, where anyone can see them? Are there multiple exits? Can they position themselves to see the door? These might seem like details, but to a traumatized nervous system scanning for threat, they're everything.

Let's start with lighting. Harsh fluorescent lights are a nervous system nightmare. They flicker at a frequency below conscious awareness but detected by neuroception. They cast sharp shadows that can trigger hypervigilance. They're often associated with institutional settings—hospitals, schools, places where many people experienced trauma. Soft, warm lighting tells the nervous system something different. It says "home" rather than "institution," "rest" rather than "alert."

Sound matters enormously. Low-frequency sounds—air conditioners, traffic, bass from music—can trigger primitive threat responses. These frequencies are similar to predator sounds in nature, and our ancient nervous systems still respond to them. High, sudden sounds trigger startle responses. Even seemingly benign sounds like phones ringing or doors slamming can shift someone out of their window of tolerance.

The physical setup of your office speaks directly to neuroception. If you're sitting behind a desk, you're creating a power differential that might trigger threat responses. If your client's back is to the door, their nervous system has to spend energy monitoring for danger from behind. If they're sitting in a chair much lower than yours, they might feel physically vulnerable. These aren't conscious thoughts—they're subcortical evaluations happening faster than awareness.

Temperature is another hidden factor. When we're cold, we naturally move toward dorsal vagal shutdown—conserving energy, withdrawing. When we're too warm, it can trigger sympathetic activation—the body preparing to deal with environmental stress. A comfortable temperature, where the body doesn't have to work to maintain homeostasis, frees up resources for engagement and healing.

Even seemingly minor things matter. That ticking clock? It might be creating a sense of urgency or counting down to something bad. The smell of strong coffee or perfume? It might be triggering implicit memories. The color of the walls? Red can increase arousal, blue can be calming, but white might feel clinical and cold.

I learned this the hard way early in my practice. I had a client who seemed increasingly agitated in sessions, and I couldn't figure out why. Finally, she burst out that the abstract art behind my chair looked like a face screaming. Her neuroception was reading it as threat every single session. Once I moved it, her whole presentation changed. The content of our work hadn't changed, but her nervous system could finally relax enough to engage.

Increasing Cues of Safety: Environmental and Relational Factors

Now, removing danger cues is just the first step. We also need to actively provide cues of safety. This is where the magic happens, where we create an environment that actually helps regulate our clients' nervous systems.

Soft textures communicate safety to our mammalian nervous system. Think about it—what do baby mammals seek for comfort? Soft fur, warm bodies. Having soft pillows, cozy blankets, or textured fabrics available tells the nervous system "this is a place of comfort, not threat." I keep a basket of different textured items—smooth stones, soft fabric, stress balls—that clients can hold if they need grounding.

Plants in the office aren't just decoration. They literally improve air quality, but more importantly, they signal life, growth, and care. A thriving plant says someone tends to this space. Dead or dying plants? They communicate neglect or death—not what we want for safety.

The placement of objects matters too. Having tissues easily accessible but not prominently displayed says "it's okay to cry here" without the pressure that a box of tissues thrust at someone might create. Having water available says "your basic needs matter." Having a clock visible to the client says "you have control over time here."

But the most powerful environmental factor is you—your regulated nervous system, your genuine presence, your social engagement system online and available. When you're truly in ventral vagal—not performing calm but actually regulated—your physiology broadcasts safety. Your breathing is regular and full. Your face is mobile and

23

expressive. Your voice has prosody. These signals tell your client's nervous system "this person is safe" more powerfully than any words could.

Your consistency becomes a safety cue. Same chair, same time, same rituals of beginning and ending. For a nervous system that's been shaped by unpredictability and chaos, this consistency is profoundly regulating. It says "this is predictable, this is manageable, this won't suddenly change."

The Therapist's Nervous System as a Therapeutic Tool

Here's something they probably didn't teach you in graduate school: your nervous system is your most powerful therapeutic tool. Not your theoretical knowledge, not your techniques, but your capacity to maintain regulation while holding space for dysregulation. This is the heart of co-regulation, and it's how healing happens.

When a client comes in activated—in sympathetic overdrive or dorsal collapse—their nervous system is looking for regulation. If you meet their activation with your own (getting anxious because they're anxious, shutting down because they're shut down), you confirm their neuroception's evaluation of danger. But if you can maintain your ventral vagal state, something else becomes possible.

Your regulated breathing starts to influence theirs—not through conscious imitation but through unconscious entrainment. Your calm presence says to their nervous system, "Whatever is happening, it's not actually life-threatening right now." Your engaged social engagement system offers connection as an alternative to defense.

But here's the tricky part: you can't fake this. Neuroception is too smart. If you're performing calm while actually activated inside, your client's nervous system will detect the incongruence. The micro-tensions in your face, the subtle changes in your breathing, the quality of your attention—these will broadcast your actual state.

This is why your own therapy, your own healing, your own nervous system regulation isn't just self-care—it's an ethical imperative. Every trigger you haven't dealt with, every trauma you haven't processed, every activation you can't regulate limits your capacity to hold space for your clients' healing. You can only take your clients as far as you've gone yourself.

I notice my own state constantly during sessions. Am I breathing fully, or has my breath gotten shallow? Are my shoulders creeping up toward my ears? Is my attention fully present, or am I starting to drift? These aren't just observations—they're information about whether I'm resourced enough to be helpful. If I'm not, I might excuse myself for a moment, take a few deep breaths in the bathroom, shake out my body, do whatever I need to return to regulation.

Cultural Considerations in Safety Perception

What signals safety to one nervous system might signal danger to another, and culture plays a huge role in this. Eye contact is a perfect example. In many Western contexts, direct eye contact signals engagement and trustworthiness. But in some cultures, direct eye contact, especially with authority figures, is disrespectful or threatening. Forcing eye contact with someone whose nervous system reads it as threat is not therapeutic—it's retraumatizing.

Physical space and touch have enormous cultural variation. In some cultures, sitting close signals warmth and connection. In others, it's invasive and threatening. Some clients might experience a handshake as connecting, others as violating. There's no universal "right way"— there's only what feels safe to this particular nervous system shaped by this particular cultural context.

Voice volume and animation vary culturally too. What reads as engaged and present in one culture might seem aggressive or overwhelming in another. What seems calm and regulated in one context might seem disconnected or cold in another. We have to be attuned not just to universal mammalian responses but to the specific cultural programming of each nervous system.

Power dynamics and authority have cultural components that affect safety. For someone from a culture with high power distance, a therapist who's too casual might feel unsafe—the lack of clear hierarchy creates uncertainty. For someone from a more egalitarian culture, too much formality might feel distancing and cold.

Even our understanding of trauma and healing is culturally bound. In individualistic cultures, we might focus on personal autonomy and individual healing. In collectivistic cultures, healing might be understood as something that happens in community, in relationship with family and ancestors. A nervous system shaped by collectivist values might not feel safe in individual therapy—the isolation itself might be triggering.

Building a Polyvagal-Informed Practice Space

Creating a truly Polyvagal-informed practice means thinking about every aspect of your client's experience, from the first phone call to the last goodbye. It means understanding that every interaction is an opportunity to communicate safety or danger to their nervous system.

The initial contact matters. Is your voicemail warm and welcoming, or clinical and distant? Does your intake paperwork feel invasive, or does it communicate respect for boundaries? Can clients choose how they want to be contacted—phone, email, text? These choices give control, and control supports safety.

The waiting room deserves careful consideration. Is there a place to sit where someone can see the door without being immediately visible to everyone who enters? Are there options—chairs, couches, different seating areas—so people can choose what feels safe to their body? Is there something to do besides anxiously wait—books, fidget items, calming music?

The transition into the therapy space is a moment of vulnerability. How do you greet your client? Do you walk ahead of them (potentially triggering for someone who needs to see threat coming) or beside them (potentially too intimate for someone who needs space)? I usually let clients lead the way once they know where we're going, so they can control the pace and distance.

In the room itself, choices support safety. "Where would you like to sit?" rather than assigned seating. "Would you like the lights brighter or dimmer?" "Is the temperature comfortable?" These aren't just niceties—they're communications that say "your nervous system's needs matter here."

Time boundaries create safety through predictability. Starting and ending on time says "I can hold boundaries," which paradoxically makes it safer to be vulnerable. But rigid adherence to time when someone is in crisis says "the schedule matters more than you." It's a dance, reading what each nervous system needs in each moment.

How you handle money affects safety. Clear, transparent fee structures reduce uncertainty. Sliding scales acknowledge financial trauma. Not talking about money creates anxiety. Talking about it too much makes the relationship feel transactional. Again, it's about finding what each particular nervous system needs.

Even how you handle documentation matters. Taking notes while someone is sharing trauma can feel like you're more interested in recording than connecting. But never taking notes might feel like you don't care enough to remember. I often ask, "How do you feel about me taking notes?" and respect whatever answer I get.

Integration and Moving Forward

Creating safety isn't a one-time setup. It's an ongoing, dynamic process of attunement and adjustment. A client who needed lots of space initially might move toward wanting more closeness as their nervous system learns you're safe. Someone who couldn't tolerate silence might begin to find it peaceful rather than threatening.

The environment that feels safe can change day to day, season to season. Winter might require different lighting than summer. A client might need different things when they're activated versus when they're shutdown. Flexibility within consistency—that's the key.

Most importantly, remember that perfect safety isn't the goal—good enough safety is. We're not trying to eliminate all possibility of activation. We're creating enough safety that the nervous system can tolerate the activation that comes with growth and healing. It's like creating a laboratory where experiments in connection and regulation can happen.

The paradox is that by focusing so intently on safety, we make it possible to work with danger—to process trauma, to feel difficult feelings, to take relational risks. Safety isn't the opposite of growth. It's the foundation that makes growth possible. When the nervous system knows it's safe, it can finally stop protecting and start healing.

Your therapy room becomes a place where nervous systems can learn something new—that connection doesn't always lead to hurt, that vulnerability doesn't always lead to violation, that someone can truly see you and not turn away. These aren't cognitive learnings. They're embodied experiences that literally rewire the nervous system, one safe moment at a time.

Chapter 4: Clinical Assessment Tools and Techniques

The first time I tried to assess a client's nervous system state using traditional methods, I felt like I was trying to paint a portrait while wearing a blindfold. Sure, I could ask about symptoms, check off boxes on standardized forms, and document what they told me. But I was missing the whole story—the one their body was telling through micro-expressions, breathing patterns, and the subtle dance of activation and shutdown happening right in front of me.

Assessment through a Polyvagal lens changes everything. Instead of just cataloging symptoms, we're mapping a living, breathing nervous system in real time. We're tracking how it moves between states, what triggers shifts, what resources bring regulation. This isn't about putting people in diagnostic boxes—it's about understanding the unique patterns of each nervous system so we can tailor our interventions precisely.

The tools and techniques I'm about to share aren't just academic exercises. They're practical ways to see what's actually happening in your client's autonomic nervous system, moment by moment. Some involve technology and formal measures. Others are as simple as noticing where someone's eyes go when they're scared. But all of them give us information we can't get any other way—information that directly guides how we help each person find their way back to safety and connection.

Standardized Polyvagal Assessment Scales and Measures

The field of Polyvagal assessment is relatively young, but we're developing increasingly sophisticated ways to measure autonomic states. The Body Perception Questionnaire, originally developed to assess body awareness, has been adapted to track the physical sensations associated with different autonomic states. Clients rate sensations like "racing heart," "heavy limbs," or "disconnection from body"—each pointing to different places on the autonomic ladder.

The Autonomic Nervous System Questionnaire takes a different approach, asking about behaviors and experiences that correlate with each state. Questions like "I find myself constantly checking doors and windows" suggest sympathetic hypervigilance, while "I often feel like I'm watching my life from outside my body" points to dorsal vagal dissociation. What makes this tool particularly useful is that it doesn't require clients to understand Polyvagal Theory—they just report their experiences.

The Safe and Sound Protocol Assessment, developed alongside Porges' listening intervention, evaluates auditory processing and social engagement. It looks at things like sensitivity to sound, ability to filter background noise, and comfort with human voice frequencies. These might seem unrelated to trauma, but they're actually windows into how the middle ear muscles—part of the social engagement system—are functioning.

But here's what I've learned: formal assessments are just starting points. The real gold comes from teaching clients to become their own assessors. I use what I call the "State Check-In"—a simple tool where clients rate themselves on three scales throughout the day: ventral (safe and social), sympathetic (activated/anxious), and dorsal (shutdown/numb). Each scale goes from 0-10, and clients can be high on more than one—you can be simultaneously activated AND shutting down, which is actually quite common in trauma.

One powerful assessment approach involves having clients identify their "home state"—where their nervous system spends most of its time. Some people live primarily in sympathetic activation, always ready for the next threat. Others default to dorsal shutdown, disconnected and numb. Still others might oscillate wildly between states, never finding solid ground. Knowing someone's home state tells us where to start our work.

I also use somatic markers as assessment tools. Where does this person hold tension? How do they breathe—shallow and quick, or barely at all? What's their baseline arousal level? These body-based assessments often tell us more than any questionnaire because the body doesn't lie. A client might tell me they're fine while their shoulders are up by their ears and they're breathing like they just ran a marathon.

Mapping Individual Nervous System Patterns and Responses

Every nervous system has its own unique signature, shaped by genetics, early experiences, trauma, and countless daily interactions. Mapping these individual patterns is like learning to read a new language—one written in breath patterns, muscle tension, and eye movements.

I start by creating what I call an "Autonomic Map" with each client. We identify what each state looks and feels like for them specifically. Sarah's sympathetic state involves leg bouncing, nail biting, and rapid speech. Tom's looks like pacing, jaw clenching, and an inability to sit still. Maria's includes a flushed face, loud voice, and aggressive gestures. Same state, completely different presentations.

Then we map triggers—what sends this particular nervous system into defense? For some, it's crowds. For others, silence. Some people are triggered by authority figures, others by peers. The triggers are as unique as fingerprints, often surprising both me and the client. I had one client who discovered that the smell of lavender—supposedly calming—sent her into immediate dorsal shutdown because her abuser wore lavender perfume.

We also map resources—what brings this nervous system back to regulation? This is where things get really interesting. Traditional self-care advice might say "take a bath" or "practice deep breathing," but those might be terrible advice for someone whose trauma involved water or suffocation. Instead, we find what actually works for this specific nervous system. Maybe it's heavy metal music, or organizing drawers, or watching cooking shows. There's no universal prescription.

Movement patterns tell us a lot about nervous system states. Someone in sympathetic activation might have jerky, quick movements or visible tension. Dorsal shutdown often shows up as slow, minimal movement or a kind of heaviness. Ventral vagal state usually involves fluid, purposeful movement with good coordination. I watch how clients move through my office, how they sit, how they gesture. It's all information.

Relational patterns are part of the map too. How does this nervous system respond to closeness versus distance? What happens when someone makes eye contact? How do they react to touch, to silence, to emotional expression? These patterns, shaped by attachment history and trauma, tell us how to calibrate our therapeutic approach.

Heart Rate Variability and Vagal Tone Assessment

Heart rate variability (HRV) is like a window into the autonomic nervous system. It measures the variation in time between heartbeats, and contrary to what you might think, more variability is actually better. It means your nervous system is flexible, responsive, able to speed up and slow down as needed. Low HRV suggests a nervous system that's rigid, stuck, unable to adapt.

Modern technology has made HRV assessment accessible. Clients can use smartphone apps paired with chest straps or finger sensors to track their HRV throughout the day. This gives us objective data about their autonomic state—not just how they think they feel, but how their nervous system is actually functioning. It's particularly useful for clients who are disconnected from their body sensations.

Respiratory sinus arrhythmia (RSA) is a specific component of HRV that's directly related to vagal tone. When we breathe in, our heart rate naturally speeds up. When we breathe out, it slows down. The bigger this difference, the better our vagal tone—the stronger our ventral vagal brake. We can actually see someone's capacity for regulation in this simple physiological measure.

I often use HRV biofeedback in sessions. Clients can watch their HRV in real time while we try different interventions. Deep breathing, visualization, movement—we can see immediately what actually shifts their nervous system toward better regulation. It's incredibly empowering for clients to see that they can influence their autonomic state, that they're not at the mercy of their nervous system.

But technology isn't always necessary. I teach clients to assess their own vagal tone through simple observations. Can they take a full, deep breath? Does their exhale naturally extend longer than their inhale? Can they sigh with relief? These simple acts require decent vagal tone. If someone can't access these basic functions, we know their ventral vagal brake is offline.

The pattern of HRV throughout the day tells us about autonomic flexibility. A healthy nervous system shows variation—higher HRV during rest, lower during activity or stress, then returning to baseline. But trauma survivors often show flattened patterns—either consistently low HRV (stuck in defense) or chaotic swings without clear patterns (dysregulated).

Creating Personal Nervous System Maps with Clients

One of the most powerful things we can do is help clients create their own personal nervous system map. This isn't something we do to them or for them—it's something we do together, making their autonomic patterns visible and understandable.

I use a simple three-ladder diagram. The top rung is ventral vagal—safe and social. The middle is sympathetic—mobilized and activated. The bottom is dorsal vagal—shutdown and withdrawn. But here's where it gets personal: we fill in what each state specifically looks like for this individual client.

For the ventral vagal state, we might note: "Can laugh easily, shoulders relaxed, breathing is full, can concentrate on reading, enjoys music, reaches out to friends." For sympathetic: "Leg bouncing, scanning for exits, irritable with family, can't eat, everything feels urgent, Netflix on but can't focus." For dorsal: "Can't get out of bed, world feels gray, nothing matters, can't cry even when sad, feel like a ghost."

Then we add triggers and glimmers. Triggers are what shift us down the ladder—from ventral to sympathetic, or from sympathetic to dorsal. Glimmers are what help us climb back up—tiny moments of safety or connection that bring regulation. We might discover that morning coffee is a glimmer that helps transition from dorsal to ventral. Or that checking work email is a trigger that launches straight into sympathetic.

The map becomes a living document. Clients take it home, add to it, notice patterns. They might realize they always go dorsal on Sunday nights (anticipating Monday) or that talking to their sister is a reliable ventral vagal anchor. The map makes the invisible visible, the unconscious conscious.

I encourage clients to share their maps with trusted people. Partners, friends, therapists—anyone who could benefit from understanding their patterns. It's amazing how relationship conflicts decrease when someone can say, "I'm in sympathetic right now, I need 10 minutes to regulate before we talk" instead of just being reactive and angry.

Tracking Autonomic State Shifts in Session

The real art of Polyvagal assessment happens in real time, tracking the subtle shifts that occur moment to moment in session. This isn't about taking notes while someone talks—it's about developing dual awareness, simultaneously present with the content and attuned to the autonomic dance.

I watch for the obvious signs first. Posture changes—someone who was leaning forward suddenly pulls back (possible shift to sympathetic). Breathing patterns—from full to shallow, or from regular to held. Eye contact—engaged to averted, or soft to intense. These are the billboard advertisements of state changes.

But the subtle signs are equally important. The quality of someone's voice might shift—losing prosody as they move toward dorsal, or becoming pressured as sympathetic kicks in. Skin tone changes—flushing with activation, or going pale with shutdown. Even the speed of speech gives us information—racing thoughts suggest sympathetic, while long pauses might indicate dorsal.

I track my own state changes too. If I suddenly feel sleepy while a client is talking about their mother, I wonder if their nervous system is pulling me into dorsal. If I feel agitated or want to interrupt, maybe their sympathetic activation is triggering mine. My nervous system becomes a sensing instrument for theirs.

Transitions are particularly revealing. How does someone's state shift when we move from casual chat to trauma content? What happens when I lean forward versus lean back? How do they respond to silence versus active engagement? These transition moments show us the edges of their window of tolerance.

I've learned to name state shifts as they happen, gently and without judgment. "I notice your breathing just changed—what are you aware of?" or "Something just shifted in your body—can you feel it?" This helps clients develop their own awareness and creates a shared language for what's happening between us.

The Art of Ongoing Assessment

Assessment isn't something we do once at the beginning of treatment. It's a continuous process, happening every moment we're with a client. Their nervous system is constantly communicating—through posture, breath, movement, voice. Our job is to become fluent in reading these signals and helping our clients read them too.

The beauty of Polyvagal assessment is that it's inherently collaborative. We're not the experts diagnosing from on high—we're partners in discovery, learning together how this particular nervous system works. Clients become scientists of their own experience, gathering data, noticing patterns, making connections.

This approach also normalizes the trauma response. Instead of "What's wrong with me?" the question becomes "What is my nervous system protecting me from?" Instead of pathology, we see adaptation. Instead of resistance, we see wisdom. This shift alone can begin to dissolve the shame that keeps so many people stuck.

As you develop these assessment skills, be patient with yourself. It takes time to develop the dual awareness needed to track content and autonomic states simultaneously. Start with one thing—maybe just breathing patterns—and gradually expand your awareness. Your nervous system needs to stay regulated enough to accurately read others, so your own regulation matters here too.

Most importantly, hold all assessments lightly. Nervous systems are dynamic, constantly changing in response to internal and external conditions. What's true today might not be true tomorrow. The map is not the territory—it's just a tool to help us navigate together toward greater regulation and resilience.

Chapter 5: Understanding Individual Autonomic Profiles

Marcus walks into my office carrying his nervous system story in every movement. His shoulders are perpetually raised, like he's bracing for impact. His eyes dart to every corner before he sits— always the same chair, always positioned so he can see the door. When he finally settles, it's more like a temporary ceasefire than actual relaxation. Without saying a word, his body has already told me volumes about where he lives on the autonomic ladder.

Every nervous system tells a unique story. Some shout their trauma history through constant mobilization. Others whisper it through profound stillness. Some oscillate wildly between extremes, never finding solid ground. Learning to read these individual patterns—to understand the specific language of each nervous system—is both an art and a science.

What I've discovered over years of practice is that there's no universal trauma response, no one-size-fits-all pattern of dysregulation. Each nervous system develops its own strategies, its own default settings, its own ways of trying to stay safe in a world that once wasn't. Understanding these individual profiles is the key to effective treatment. We're not treating "trauma"—we're working with this specific nervous system, shaped by these particular experiences, trying to find its unique path back to regulation.

Identifying Triggers and Glimmers for Each Autonomic State

Triggers and glimmers are the switches that move us up and down the autonomic ladder. But here's what's fascinating—what triggers one person might be neutral or even regulating for another. The smell of coffee might bring one client into pleasant ventral vagal morning ritual, while sending another straight into sympathetic activation because their abusive parent always smelled like coffee during morning rages.

I work with clients to become detectives of their own nervous system. We start with obvious triggers—the ones they already know about. Loud noises, certain people, specific places. But then we go deeper, looking for the subtle triggers they might not have noticed. The way afternoon light falls through windows. The sound of keys jingling. That particular tone of voice that says someone's about to get angry.

Rachel discovered her nervous system was triggered by silence. Not conflict, not yelling—silence. Growing up, silence meant her mother was giving her the cold shoulder, punishing her with withdrawal of love. Now, thirty years later, her nervous system still reads silence as danger. Her husband's quiet morning routine, meant to let her sleep in, was actually triggering sympathetic activation before her day even started.

Glimmers are just as individual. Standard self-care advice might say "take a warm bath," but for someone whose trauma involved water, that's a trigger, not a glimmer. We need to find what actually brings this specific nervous system toward regulation. Sometimes it's surprising. I've had clients find glimmers in death metal music, organizing spreadsheets, or watching horror movies. The nervous system knows what it needs, even if it doesn't match conventional wisdom.

Micro-glimmers are particularly powerful. These are tiny moments of regulation that might last only seconds but can begin to shift an entire day. The first sip of tea. Petting a dog. The moment when a favorite song comes on the radio. We're not looking for big, dramatic shifts—we're collecting these tiny moments of ventral vagal activation like breadcrumbs leading back to safety.

I teach clients to track patterns. Does the trigger always lead to the same state? Some triggers might send them to sympathetic fight, others to sympathetic flight, still others straight to dorsal shutdown. Understanding these patterns helps predict and prepare for state shifts.

Recognizing State-Specific Behaviors and Presentations

Each autonomic state comes with its own set of behaviors, thoughts, and ways of being in the world. But how these states manifest is deeply personal, shaped by temperament, culture, trauma history, and learned coping strategies.

Take sympathetic activation. For some, it shows up as anger—raised voice, clenched fists, aggressive posturing. For others, it's anxiety—racing thoughts, catastrophizing, can't sit still. Still others might experience it as perfectionism—everything must be controlled, planned, managed. Same autonomic state, completely different presentations.

I worked with two clients, both stuck in chronic sympathetic activation. James expressed it through workaholism—80-hour weeks, constant productivity, unable to rest. "If I stop moving, something bad will happen," his nervous system believed. Lisa expressed it through hypochondria—constantly checking her body, googling symptoms, convinced something was terribly wrong. Both were in mobilization, but their behaviors looked nothing alike.

Dorsal vagal shutdown is equally variable. Some people in dorsal look obviously depressed—can't get out of bed, no energy, flat affect. But others might look functional, even successful, while being profoundly disconnected. They go through the motions, show up to work, maintain relationships, all while feeling like they're watching someone else's life through glass.

The key is learning each person's specific tells. When Mark goes into sympathetic, his speech speeds up and he starts using military terminology—everything becomes a mission, a battle, a strategic objective. When he shifts to dorsal, his voice goes flat and he starts speaking in third person, distancing himself from his own experience.

Ventral vagal presence also looks different for different people. For some, it's obviously social—chatty, engaged, reaching out to others. For others, it might be quietly creative—absorbed in art or music or writing. Some people's ventral vagal state is active and playful, others' is calm and contemplative. There's no right way to be regulated.

Story Follows State: How Autonomic States Shape Narratives

Here's something that will change how you listen to clients: the stories they tell about themselves and their lives are shaped by their current autonomic state. Same events, same history, but told from sympathetic activation versus dorsal shutdown? Completely different narrative.

When clients are in sympathetic activation, their stories tend to be about danger, betrayal, the need to fight or escape. Everyone becomes a potential threat. The future is catastrophic. The past is full of warning signs they should have seen. They might tell me about their childhood and focus entirely on the chaos, the unpredictability, the times they had to be vigilant.

Shift that same client to dorsal vagal, and the story changes. Now it's about helplessness, hopelessness, being trapped. The same childhood becomes a story of neglect, abandonment, being invisible. The future doesn't exist. The past is a gray fog of disconnection.

But get someone into ventral vagal, and watch the narrative transform again. Now they can hold complexity. Their childhood had trauma AND moments of joy. They can see how they survived, adapted, showed resilience. The future has possibilities. The present has choice.

I saw this dramatically with Elena. In sympathetic, she'd tell me how everyone at work was out to get her, how she had to fight for everything, how exhausting it was to always be on guard. In dorsal, she'd say work didn't matter, nothing she did made a difference, she was invisible and irrelevant. But on the rare days she came in regulated, she could say, "My job has challenges, but I'm good at what I do and I have some supportive colleagues."

This is why cognitive therapy alone can be so limited with trauma. We might challenge someone's "negative thoughts," but if their nervous system is in a defensive state, those thoughts are just accurately reflecting their autonomic reality. The story follows the state. Change the state, and the story naturally shifts.

Understanding this helps us hold clients' narratives more lightly. The catastrophizing isn't a cognitive distortion—it's sympathetic activation speaking. The hopelessness isn't depression—it's dorsal vagal narrating. Our job isn't to argue with these stories but to help regulate the nervous system so different stories become possible.

Assessment of Autonomic Flexibility and Resilience

Autonomic flexibility is the ability to move appropriately between states based on actual environmental demands. It's not about being in ventral vagal all the time—sometimes we need sympathetic mobilization, occasionally even dorsal withdrawal serves a purpose. Health is about being able to shift states as needed and then return to baseline.

I assess flexibility by observing how clients move between states. Can they shift smoothly, or are the transitions jarring? Can they come back to baseline after activation, or do they get stuck? How long does it take to recover from a trigger? These patterns tell us about nervous system resilience.

Some people have what I call "sticky" nervous systems—once they shift into a defensive state, they stay there for hours or days. Others have "jumpy" nervous systems—constantly shifting states, never settling anywhere. Still others have "narrow" nervous systems—they can only access a limited range of states, missing either the activation of sympathetic or the restoration of ventral vagal.

Recovery time is a key measure of resilience. A flexible nervous system might get triggered into sympathetic by a stressful email, but return to baseline within minutes. A less flexible system might stay activated all day. We track these patterns: How long does it take to come back from sympathetic activation? How long to emerge from

41

dorsal shutdown? These recovery times often improve with treatment, giving us a way to measure progress.

I also look at state-switching triggers. A resilient nervous system needs a significant threat to shift into defense. A sensitized nervous system might shift with minimal provocation. One client might need an actual dangerous situation to go sympathetic. Another might get triggered by someone walking too close at the grocery store.

Context-appropriateness matters too. Does the nervous system response match the actual situation? Getting activated during a job interview—that makes sense. Getting activated while watching TV with loved ones—that suggests the nervous system is responding to past rather than present danger.

Documentation and Treatment Planning Based on Autonomic Profiles

Traditional treatment planning focuses on symptoms and diagnoses. Polyvagal-informed treatment planning focuses on autonomic patterns and regulation strategies. We're not just trying to reduce anxiety—we're trying to increase ventral vagal access. We're not just addressing depression—we're working to mobilize out of dorsal shutdown.

I document several key elements in autonomic profiles. First, the home state—where does this nervous system spend most of its time? Second, the range—what states can they access, and which are offline? Third, triggers and glimmers for each state. Fourth, recovery patterns—how quickly can they return to baseline? Fifth, resources—what helps this specific nervous system regulate?

Treatment goals become more precise. Instead of "reduce anxiety," we might aim to "increase capacity to downregulate from sympathetic activation within 20 minutes." Instead of "improve mood," we target "develop three reliable ways to shift from dorsal to ventral vagal." These are measurable, achievable, and directly connected to autonomic functioning.

The treatment plan includes state-specific interventions. For sympathetic activation: vigorous movement to discharge energy, cold water on the face to trigger the dive response, bilateral stimulation to integrate activation. For dorsal shutdown: gentle movement to create mobilization, rhythm and music to activate, temperature changes to stimulate awareness.

We also plan for different phases of treatment. Early phase might focus on stabilization—expanding the window of tolerance, developing basic regulation skills. Middle phase might involve processing—working with trauma while maintaining enough regulation. Later phase emphasizes integration—building autonomic flexibility and resilience for daily life.

The autonomic profile informs the therapeutic approach itself. A client stuck in dorsal needs a different presence than one in chronic sympathetic. With dorsal, I might be more actively engaging, using more prosody in my voice, more animation in my face—lending them my ventral vagal activation. With sympathetic, I might be calmer, slower, more grounded—offering my regulation as an anchor.

Building a Complete Picture

Understanding individual autonomic profiles transforms how we work. We stop trying to fit people into diagnostic boxes and start working with their unique nervous system patterns. We stop applying generic interventions and start tailoring our approach to what this specific nervous system needs.

The profile isn't fixed—it's a living document that evolves as the nervous system heals. Early in treatment, someone might have a very narrow window, limited state access, and long recovery times. As we work together, the window expands, new states come online, resilience builds. The profile helps us track this progress in concrete, observable ways.

This approach also empowers clients. Instead of feeling at the mercy of mysterious symptoms, they understand their patterns. They can predict triggers, recognize state shifts, and apply appropriate interventions. They become experts in their own nervous system, which is exactly where the expertise belongs.

Most importantly, understanding autonomic profiles helps us work with, not against, the nervous system's wisdom. Every pattern developed for a reason. Every default state once served survival. By respecting these adaptations while gently introducing new possibilities, we honor both the trauma and the healing.

As you develop skill in recognizing autonomic profiles, you'll find yourself naturally attuning to the subtle differences in each nervous system. You'll stop asking "What's wrong?" and start asking "What happened?" You'll stop seeing pathology and start seeing adaptation. And in that shift, everything changes—for you and for your clients.

Chapter 6: The Science and Art of Co-Regulation

Two nervous systems sit in my office. Mine, ideally regulated and present. My client's, often defensive and guarded. What happens between us in the next fifty minutes isn't just conversation—it's a biological dance of neural communication that happens mostly below conscious awareness. Our nervous systems are talking to each other in a language older than words, negotiating safety, testing trust, seeking connection.

Co-regulation isn't a technique you apply—it's something that happens naturally when two nervous systems meet. The question isn't whether we're co-regulating with our clients. We always are. The question is whether we're doing it consciously, skillfully, and in service of healing. Because make no mistake: your nervous system is either a resource for your client's regulation or another source of dysregulation.

This is why therapy is both science and art. The science tells us how nervous systems communicate, what signals create safety, how regulation spreads from one person to another. The art is in the moment-to-moment attunement, the subtle adjustments, the exquisite sensitivity to when to lean in and when to give space. It's jazz, not classical music—structured improvisation based on deep knowledge but expressed through intuitive presence.

Co-Regulation as Reciprocal Safety Signaling Between Nervous Systems

Co-regulation starts before anyone speaks. When your client walks in, their nervous system is already evaluating yours. Are you genuinely present or distracted? Is your breathing calm or stressed? Is your face open or guarded? These assessments happen through neuroception, faster than conscious thought, and they determine whether your client's nervous system decides you're safe enough for vulnerability.

Think about how mammals in the wild establish safety. They don't exchange credentials or discuss boundaries. They read each other's nervous systems through posture, movement, breath, and facial expression. A calm animal with soft eyes and relaxed body signals safety. A tense animal with darting eyes signals danger. We're not so different. Despite our complex language and abstract thinking, our mammalian nervous systems still communicate primarily through these ancient channels.

The reciprocal nature of co-regulation is crucial. It's not just me regulating you or you regulating me—it's a continuous feedback loop. My calm presence might help settle your activation, which allows you to access more social engagement, which signals safety back to me, which helps me stay even more regulated. It's a upward spiral of mutual regulation, each nervous system supporting the other.

But the opposite is equally true. If I'm activated—stressed about my schedule, worried about a personal issue, frustrated with a previous client—my nervous system broadcasts danger. Your already defensive nervous system picks this up and becomes more guarded. You sense my activation and shut down further. I notice your withdrawal and become more anxious about the session. Now we're in a downward spiral of mutual dysregulation.

This is why your own regulation isn't just self-care—it's the foundation of effective therapy. Every time you walk into a session dysregulated, you're asking your client's nervous system to work harder, to overcome not just their own defensive patterns but also the danger signals coming from you. It's like trying to teach someone to swim while you're drowning.

The signals we exchange are multimodal. Vocal prosody—the music of our voice—carries enormous information about our state. A flat, monotonous voice signals dorsal withdrawal. A pressured, harsh voice signals sympathetic activation. A melodic, varied voice signals ventral vagal safety. Our nervous systems are exquisitely tuned to these vocal qualities, reading safety or danger in the space between words.

Nonverbal Cues and the Social Engagement System

The social engagement system is our biological equipment for connection, linking heart regulation with the muscles of social communication. When this system is online, we naturally produce and read the nonverbal cues that create safety between nervous systems. But trauma often compromises this system, making both sending and receiving these cues difficult.

Facial expression is primary. Our faces have more muscles than any other body part precisely because facial communication is so crucial for mammals. A genuine smile—not just mouth but also eyes—signals ventral vagal state. Soft eyes with slightly raised eyebrows communicate openness and interest. But a frozen face, even if smiling, signals danger. The nervous system knows the difference between authentic and performed expressions.

Eye contact is complex territory. The right amount of eye contact—soft, intermittent, responsive—facilitates co-regulation. But too much becomes intrusive, triggering defensive responses. Too little signals disinterest or danger. And for many trauma survivors, any eye contact feels threatening because their social engagement system associates being seen with being hurt.

I learned to let clients lead with eye contact. I make it available—my gaze soft and open—but don't demand it. When they look away, I might too, reducing the intensity. When they look back, I'm there, available but not overwhelming. It's a dance of connection and space, always respecting their nervous system's needs.

Head position and movement matter more than most people realize. The way we tilt our head signals whether we're listening (slight tilt) or challenging (chin up). Nodding isn't just agreement—it's a co-regulatory behavior that says "I'm with you, we're in sync." But mechanical nodding without genuine attunement feels false and breaks co-regulation.

Physical distance and orientation create different co-regulatory fields. Sitting directly across from someone can feel confrontational to a defensive nervous system. Sitting at an angle allows for connection with less intensity. Too close triggers threat; too far signals disconnection. The sweet spot varies for each nervous system, and it can change even within a single session.

The Therapist's Embodied Awareness and Regulation

Your body is your instrument in this work. Just as a violinist must keep their instrument tuned, you must maintain awareness of your own nervous system state. This isn't narcissistic navel-gazing—it's professional responsibility. Your regulated presence is often the most powerful intervention you can offer.

I start each day with a body scan. Where am I holding tension? How's my breathing? What's my overall activation level? This baseline awareness helps me notice shifts throughout the day. If I'm getting progressively more activated with each client, I know I need to regulate between sessions. If I'm sliding toward dorsal shutdown by afternoon, I need mobilization.

Between sessions, even just two minutes of regulation can make a difference. I might step outside and feel sunlight on my face (ventral vagal activation). Or do some gentle stretching (proprioceptive input that supports regulation). Or listen to a favorite song (auditory regulation). These aren't breaks—they're essential maintenance of my therapeutic instrument.

During sessions, I maintain dual awareness—tracking both my client's state and my own. If I notice my shoulders creeping up, I gently release them. If my breathing gets shallow, I consciously deepen it. If I'm leaning forward with too much intensity, I settle back. These micro-regulations happen continuously, below my client's conscious awareness but detected by their neuroception.

But here's the tricky part: authentic regulation can't be performed. You can't fake a calm nervous system. If you're trying to appear calm while actually activated inside, the incongruence creates confusion and mistrust. Better to acknowledge, "I'm noticing I'm a bit activated by what you're sharing. Let me take a breath so I can really be present with you." This honesty actually builds safety—it shows you're human and that you're taking responsibility for your own regulation.

Eight Essential Co-Regulation Skills for Therapeutic Relationships

Over years of practice, I've identified eight core skills that facilitate co-regulation. These aren't techniques to apply mechanically but capacities to develop and refine.

1. Attuned Presence: This is more than just being in the room. It's bringing your full attention, your whole nervous system, into resonance with your client. It means putting aside your agenda, your theories, your need to help, and just being with what is. When clients feel truly met in this way, their nervous system can begin to relax its vigilance.

2. Regulatory Flexibility: The ability to adjust your own state in response to your client's needs. With someone in dorsal shutdown, you might need to bring more activation—more animation in your voice, more movement in your body. With someone in sympathetic overdrive, you become an anchor of calm. This isn't about matching their state but offering the complementary regulation they need.

3. Prosodic Range: Your voice is a powerful co-regulatory tool. Learning to consciously use pitch, rhythm, volume, and tone to communicate safety and engagement. A sing-song quality can help regulate an anxious nervous system. A slightly lower pitch can ground someone who's dissociating. The music of your voice often matters more than the words.

4. Somatic Awareness: Knowing what's happening in your body moment to moment and using that information. If you suddenly feel

49

sleepy, it might be your client's dorsal state pulling you down. If you feel agitated, you might be picking up their sympathetic activation. This somatic countertransference is valuable information about what's happening between your nervous systems.

5. Boundary Flexibility: Knowing when to lean in and when to create space. Some moments call for increased proximity and intensity of connection. Others require backing off, reducing demand. This isn't based on rules but on reading what each nervous system needs in each moment.

6. Rupture Repair: Co-regulation inevitably breaks. You misattune, say the wrong thing, trigger a defensive response. The ability to recognize ruptures quickly and repair them is essential. "I think I just missed you there. Can we back up?" This repair actually strengthens co-regulation by showing that connection can be broken and restored.

7. State Naming: The ability to gently name autonomic states as they arise. "I notice your breathing just changed." "Something just shifted in your body." "I'm sensing you might be moving toward shutdown." This helps clients develop awareness and also shows that you're tracking them closely, which paradoxically increases safety.

8. Transitional Attunement: Being sensitive to the transitions—beginning and end of session, shifting between topics, moving from casual to deeper material. These transition moments are when nervous systems are most vulnerable. Slowing down, explicitly marking transitions, checking in about readiness—these all support maintained co-regulation.

Managing Therapeutic Ruptures Through Co-Regulatory Repair

Ruptures in co-regulation aren't failures—they're opportunities. Every relationship involves misattunement, disconnection, moments where nervous systems fall out of sync. What matters isn't preventing ruptures but how we repair them.

A rupture might be obvious—you say something that triggers your client, they shut down or get angry. Or it might be subtle—a slight withdrawal, a change in breathing, a loss of eye contact. The key is catching ruptures quickly, before they compound into bigger disconnections.

When I notice a rupture, I first regulate myself. If I get anxious about the disconnection and rush to fix it, I'll likely make things worse. A breath, a moment to ground myself, then I can address what happened. "Something just shifted between us. Can you help me understand what just happened for you?"

Sometimes the rupture is my fault—I misattuned, made an assumption, pushed too hard. Acknowledging this directly is powerful: "I think I just moved too fast there. I'm sorry. Can we slow down?" This models accountability and shows that the relationship can tolerate honesty about mistakes.

Other times, the rupture comes from the client's nervous system detecting danger that isn't there—a trigger from past trauma, a misread signal. Here, gentle exploration helps: "I noticed you just pulled back. Did something I said land wrong?" We're not looking for blame but understanding what each nervous system experienced.

Repair requires both nervous systems to be regulated enough to reconnect. If your client is in full sympathetic activation or dorsal shutdown, immediate repair might not be possible. First, we need to help their nervous system return to a state where connection is possible. Then we can explore what happened.

The beautiful thing about successful repair is that it actually strengthens co-regulation. It teaches both nervous systems that connection can be disrupted and restored, that relationships can survive imperfection, that safety can be rebuilt. For clients whose early relationships involved ruptures without repair, this can be profoundly healing.

The Dance of Two Nervous Systems

Co-regulation is happening whether we're conscious of it or not. Every moment in the therapy room, two nervous systems are negotiating, communicating, influencing each other. By bringing awareness and skill to this process, we can use it intentionally in service of healing.

This work requires us to be instruments of regulation, which means tending to our own nervous system with the same care we bring to our clients'. It means developing sensitivity to the subtle signals of safety and danger we're broadcasting. It means being willing to be changed by the encounter, to let our nervous system be touched by another's pain and resilience.

The science gives us the map—understanding how nervous systems communicate, what signals create safety, how regulation spreads between bodies. But the art is in the implementation—the moment-to-moment attunement, the delicate dance of connection and space, the intuitive sense of what this particular nervous system needs in this particular moment.

As you develop these co-regulatory skills, be patient with yourself. This is embodied learning that happens over time, through practice and reflection. Your nervous system needs to learn these patterns just as much as your cognitive mind. And remember—perfect co-regulation isn't the goal. Good enough co-regulation, with rupture and repair, is where healing happens.

Chapter 7: Advanced Co-Regulation Techniques

The moment Maria walked into my office, I knew something was different. Not because of what she said—she hadn't spoken yet. Her nervous system was broadcasting a new state, something between the familiar collapse I'd seen for months and actual engagement. Her voice, when she finally spoke, had a hint of melody that hadn't been there before. "I tried that thing we talked about," she said, "humming when I feel myself going away. It's weird, but it works."

Advanced co-regulation isn't about fancy techniques or complicated interventions. It's about understanding the subtle channels through which nervous systems communicate and learning to use them intentionally. Your voice becomes a tuning fork. Your movements create a rhythm others can sync with. Your regulated presence becomes a bridge back to connection for nervous systems that have forgotten how to trust.

What I'm about to share goes beyond basic co-regulation. These are the refined skills that come from understanding how specific elements—prosody, rhythm, movement, even silence—can be used therapeutically. These aren't party tricks. They're precise interventions based on how mammalian nervous systems actually connect and communicate.

Vocal Prosody and Facial Expression in Therapy

Your voice is doing way more than carrying words. The musical qualities of your voice—the rise and fall, the rhythm, the tone—speak directly to your client's nervous system in a language older than speech. Prosody, that sing-song quality of engaged conversation, is actually a marker of ventral vagal activation. When we're safe and social, our voice naturally has more melody. When we're defensive, it flattens or becomes harsh.

I discovered this accidentally with Tom, a veteran who could barely speak above a monotone. Everything he said sounded like a military report—flat, factual, devoid of emotion. One day, I consciously exaggerated the prosody in my own voice, not mockingly, but genuinely increasing the musical quality. Within minutes, his voice began to shift. Tiny variations appeared. By the end of the session, there were actual inflections. His nervous system was borrowing my prosody to remember its own capacity for vocal expression.

The specific frequencies matter too. Higher frequencies (though not shrill) tend to signal safety to our nervous system. This is why we instinctively use higher pitches when talking to babies or frightened animals. Lower frequencies, especially sudden low sounds, can trigger threat responses. But a warm, steady low tone can be grounding for someone who's dissociating—it provides an anchor.

Rhythm in speech creates predictability, which supports regulation. Not robotic rhythm, but the natural cadence of engaged conversation. When someone's in sympathetic activation, speaking slightly slower than their rapid pace can help their nervous system downshift. When they're in dorsal shutdown, matching their slow pace initially, then gradually increasing, can help mobilize them.

Facial expressions are equally powerful. Our brains have specialized neurons dedicated to reading faces, and trauma often disrupts this system. A frozen therapeutic face, even if professionally neutral, can trigger threat responses. But overdoing expressions can feel false or overwhelming. The key is authentic, responsive facial mobility that matches the emotional tone of what's being discussed.

The eyes are particularly important. Soft eyes with slightly raised eyebrows communicate openness and safety. But sustained eye contact can be threatening. I use what I call "available gaze"—my eyes are soft and available, but I also look away naturally, reducing

54

intensity. When clients look away, I often do too, then return when they return. It's a dance of connection and space.

Micro-expressions matter more than you might think. That tiny furrow of concentration when you're listening, the slight smile when they share something positive, the concerned eyebrow raise when they describe pain—these small movements signal that you're present, that you're tracking them, that they matter. Clients might not consciously notice, but their neuroception is reading every signal.

Rhythmic Movement and Synchronization Techniques

Movement and rhythm are fundamental to regulation. Think about how we naturally rock babies, how we tap our feet to music, how walking can calm anxiety. These aren't just habits—they're our nervous system using rhythm and movement to regulate. In therapy, we can use these same principles intentionally.

Bilateral stimulation doesn't require fancy equipment. Simply having clients tap alternately on their knees, or cross their arms and tap their shoulders, creates a rhythmic, bilateral pattern that can help integrate activation. The key is finding the right pace—too fast increases activation, too slow might not engage the nervous system enough. I let clients find their own rhythm, then we adjust from there.

Walking therapy, when possible, naturally creates bilateral stimulation and rhythm. Side-by-side movement also reduces the intensity of face-to-face interaction, making it easier for some clients to access difficult material. The shared rhythm of walking together creates a kind of embodied co-regulation that's different from sitting still.

Even in a traditional office setting, we can use subtle movement. Gentle rocking in a chair, if available, provides vestibular input that many find regulating. Having stress balls or fidget items available gives the nervous system something to do with mobilization energy. Some clients regulate better when their hands are busy—knitting, doodling, playing with therapy putty.

55

Synchrony exercises can powerfully demonstrate co-regulation. I might have clients mirror my movements—raising arms slowly, then lowering them. Or we might breathe together, finding a shared rhythm. This isn't about perfect matching but about experiencing what it feels like when two nervous systems sync up. For clients who've never experienced safe attunement, this can be profound.

The rhythm of the session itself matters. Predictable opening rituals, consistent timing of breaks, reliable closing routines—these create a rhythm that supports regulation. I had one client who needed exactly three minutes of casual chat before we could go deeper. Less felt rushed; more felt like avoidance. Finding and honoring these rhythms is part of advanced co-regulation.

Internal Co-Regulation: Supporting Client Self-Regulation

The ultimate goal isn't for clients to need us forever—it's for them to develop their own internal co-regulation capacity. This means teaching them to be in relationship with their own nervous system the way we are with theirs: curious, compassionate, responsive.

Internal co-regulation starts with differentiation. Can clients recognize different parts of their internal experience? There's the part that's scared, the part that's angry, the part that wants to shut down, and crucially, the part that can observe all these other parts. This observing self—what some call the "witness"—is the internal co-regulator.

I teach clients to have internal dialogues with their nervous system. "Okay, nervous system, I can feel you getting activated. What do you need right now?" This isn't dissociation—it's developing a relationship with their own physiological state. They're learning to be the regulated presence for their own dysregulated states.

Imagery can support internal co-regulation. Some clients imagine their ventral vagal self as a warm, golden light that can spread through their body. Others picture their regulated self as a wise, calm presence that can comfort activated parts. One client imagined her regulated self as a strong tree that could shelter her frightened inner child. The specific image doesn't matter—what matters is creating an internal resource for co-regulation.

Self-touch is a powerful form of internal co-regulation that's often overlooked. Placing a hand on your heart, holding your own hand, wrapping your arms around yourself—these activate the same neural pathways as receiving comfort from another. But many trauma survivors have complicated relationships with touch. We work slowly, finding what kind of self-touch feels safe and regulating.

The voice can be used for internal co-regulation. Humming creates vibration that stimulates the vagus nerve. Singing, even badly, requires breath control that supports regulation. Some clients talk to themselves in soothing tones, becoming their own source of prosodic regulation. One client recorded herself reading calming passages when regulated, then listened during activation.

Group Therapy Applications and Collective Co-Regulation

Group therapy adds layers of complexity to co-regulation. Now we're not dealing with two nervous systems but multiple nervous systems all influencing each other. One person's activation can ripple through the group. But equally, the group's collective regulation can hold and stabilize someone who's struggling.

The physical setup matters enormously in groups. Circles allow everyone to see everyone, but can feel exposing. Semicircles with the therapist as anchor can feel safer. Having options—chairs, floor cushions, standing space—lets nervous systems choose what they need. I always have at least one chair near the door for those who need an escape route to feel safe.

Opening rituals are crucial for group co-regulation. We might start with a breathing exercise, everyone finding a shared rhythm. Or a simple check-in using body sensations rather than emotions: "tight chest," "heavy legs," "buzzing hands." This helps everyone arrive and gives the group a sense of where everyone's nervous system is starting.

Group contagion is real. One person's panic attack can trigger sympathetic activation throughout the room. But I've also seen profound collective regulation—the group naturally breathing together, settling together, creating a field of safety that holds everyone. The therapist's job is partly to be a stabilizing force when contagion threatens and to recognize and amplify collective regulation when it emerges.

Pairs and subgroups can practice co-regulation directly. Simple exercises like synchronized breathing, mirrored movements, or taking turns being the "regulator" and the "regulated" help members experience both sides of co-regulation. This builds capacity and also demonstrates that everyone has something to offer, regardless of their trauma history.

The group becomes a laboratory for testing co-regulation in relationships. Members learn to recognize when they're being pulled into someone else's activation, when they're broadcasting their own dysregulation, and when genuine co-regulation is happening. These are skills they can take into their daily relationships.

Telehealth Adaptations for Co-Regulatory Practices

The pandemic forced us all to figure out how to co-regulate through screens, and honestly? It's harder but not impossible. The nervous system can still read cues through video, though some channels are limited. We lose full body language, smell, and the subtle energy of physical presence. But we gain other things—clients in their own safe space, the ability to use their own resources, and sometimes less intensity, which some nervous systems prefer.

Screen placement makes a huge difference. Having the camera at eye level creates better facial visibility. Being too close can feel intrusive; too far makes facial expressions hard to read. I coach clients on finding the sweet spot where we can see each other's faces clearly but not feel overwhelmed by the screen presence.

Audio quality matters more in telehealth. Poor audio creates stress for the nervous system—we're straining to hear, missing prosodic cues, dealing with delays. Investing in good microphones and encouraging clients to use headphones improves the co-regulatory channel of voice. Sometimes closing video and focusing solely on voice creates better connection than poor-quality video.

Explicit naming becomes more important online. "I'm noticing I can't quite read your expression—can you tell me what's happening for you?" or "I'm aware we're missing some of the usual cues we'd have in person—let's check in more frequently." This acknowledgment itself can help regulate the frustration of limited connection.

Screen fatigue is real and affects co-regulation. The nervous system works harder to read cues through video, which can lead to faster dysregulation. Shorter sessions, more breaks, or phone sessions interspersed with video can help. Some clients regulate better with video off, just voice connection. Others need the visual. There's no one right way.

Creative adaptations can enhance online co-regulation. Having clients place a hand on their heart while the therapist does the same creates a shared somatic experience. Using screenshare to look at calming images together, or having synchronized breathing with a visual guide, can strengthen co-regulation despite the distance.

The Refinement of Connection

Advanced co-regulation techniques aren't about doing something to clients—they're about refining our capacity to be with clients in ways that support their nervous system's journey back to connection. Every element—our voice, our face, our movements, even our presence through a screen—becomes part of the therapeutic instrument.

These techniques require practice and sensitivity. What works for one nervous system might be overwhelming or insufficient for another.

The art is in the attunement—reading what this particular nervous system needs in this particular moment and adjusting accordingly. Sometimes that means amplifying your prosody; sometimes it means being very still. Sometimes it means perfect synchrony; sometimes it means gentle differentiation.

As you develop these advanced skills, remember that perfect co-regulation isn't the goal. We're not trying to create dependency on our regulation but to offer experiences that help clients remember and rebuild their own capacity for connection. Every moment of successful co-regulation is teaching their nervous system that connection is possible, that others can be safe, that they can both receive and offer regulation.

The beauty of this work is that it changes us too. As we refine our co-regulatory skills, our own nervous systems become more flexible, more resilient. We learn to maintain regulation in the face of others' dysregulation, to offer stability without rigidity, to be affected without being overwhelmed. This isn't just professional development—it's personal growth at the deepest level.

Chapter 8: Understanding and Assessing the Window of Tolerance

Jennifer sits across from me, describing her week with increasing agitation. "Monday was fine, Tuesday was okay, but then Wednesday—I don't know what happened. My boss asked a simple question and suddenly I couldn't think, couldn't speak. I just shut down. Then later I exploded at my partner over nothing. I feel like I'm either numb or on fire, nothing in between." She's describing what happens when life pushes us outside our window of tolerance—that zone where we can handle stress without losing our ability to function.

Dan Siegel's concept of the window of tolerance gives us a perfect framework for understanding how trauma affects our capacity to stay regulated. Think of it as your nervous system's comfort zone—the space where you can experience emotions, think clearly, and respond rather than react. For some people, this window is wide and flexible. They can handle significant stress while staying relatively centered. For trauma survivors, this window often becomes narrow and rigid, with even minor stressors pushing them into chaos or rigidity.

What makes this concept so clinically useful is how perfectly it maps onto Polyvagal Theory. Your window of tolerance is essentially your ventral vagal range—the zone where your social engagement system stays online. Push beyond the upper edge, and you're in sympathetic hyperarousal. Fall below the lower edge, and you're in dorsal hypoarousal. Understanding this helps both therapists and clients visualize what's happening in the nervous system and, more importantly, what to do about it.

Dan Siegel's Window of Tolerance Model and Polyvagal Integration

When Siegel introduced the window of tolerance concept, he gave us a visual metaphor that makes autonomic states understandable to anyone. Inside the window, we're in what he calls the "river of integration"—thoughts and feelings flow, we can reflect on experiences, we stay connected to ourselves and others. This maps perfectly onto the ventral vagal state that Porges describes, where our social engagement system keeps us regulated and connected.

The upper edge of the window is the threshold into hyperarousal— what Siegel calls the "chaos" zone. Here, emotions flood us, thoughts race, impulses take over. In Polyvagal terms, we've shifted into sympathetic activation. The nervous system has decided there's danger and mobilized for action. We might experience anxiety, panic, rage, or overwhelming urgency. Everything speeds up and intensifies.

The lower edge leads to hypoarousal—Siegel's "rigidity" zone. Here, we go numb, disconnect, can't think or feel properly. This is dorsal vagal territory, where the nervous system has decided the threat is too overwhelming to fight or flee, so it shuts down. Time seems to stop or becomes meaningless. We might feel empty, absent, or like we're watching life from very far away.

What's brilliant about this model is how it shows that both extremes— chaos and rigidity—are outside our optimal functioning zone. Many people think of trauma responses as just being "too activated" and miss the shutdown piece. Or they pathologize their numbness without understanding it's just the flip side of hyperarousal. Both are defensive states, both are protective, and both take us out of our window where healing and growth happen.

The window isn't fixed. It fluctuates based on numerous factors—how much sleep you got, what you ate, whether you feel supported, the time of year, hormonal cycles, current stressors. I've had clients track their window over time and discover patterns. One woman noticed her window narrowed dramatically the week before her period. Another realized his window was widest on days he exercised in the morning.

Trauma significantly narrows the window. When your nervous system has learned that the world is dangerous, it keeps you closer to the edges, ready to tip into defense at any moment. Some trauma survivors have such narrow windows they're constantly bouncing between hyperarousal and hypoarousal, never finding solid ground in between. They might wake up anxious, crash into numbness by noon, spike back to panic by evening. It's exhausting.

Hyperarousal and Hypoarousal: Clinical Presentations

Hyperarousal looks different in different people, but the underlying physiology is the same—sympathetic nervous system overdrive. Some people experience it primarily as anxiety: racing thoughts, catastrophic thinking, can't sit still, checking locks repeatedly. Others experience it as anger: irritability, rage, looking for fights, everything feels like an attack. Still others might experience it somatically: racing heart, sweating, digestive issues, muscle tension.

In session, hyperaroused clients might talk rapidly, interrupt, seem unable to track what you're saying. They might fidget constantly, scan the room, startle at small sounds. Their breathing is often shallow and rapid. They might report insomnia, nightmares, or waking up already activated. Everything feels urgent, like there's no time, like something terrible is about to happen.

I worked with Marcus, whose hyperarousal presented as hypervigilance and control. He had contingency plans for contingency plans. Every conversation was a strategic assessment of threat. He couldn't relax because relaxing meant dropping his guard, and dropping his guard meant danger. His window of tolerance was so narrow that even positive surprises—unexpected good news—would push him into activation.

Hypoarousal is often missed or misdiagnosed because it can look like calm from the outside. But inside, the person is gone—disconnected, numb, unable to feel or think properly. Some describe it as being behind glass, underwater, or floating above their body. Others say it's like the world lost its color, like nothing matters, like they're already dead.

In therapy, hypoaroused clients might seem spacey, forget what they were saying mid-sentence, or stare blankly. Their voice often goes flat, monotonous. They might report sleeping too much but never feeling rested, or being unable to cry even when they desperately want to. Time distortion is common—sessions feel like they last forever or pass in an instant.

Sarah would arrive for sessions looking functional, even put-together. But when she tried to access emotions about her trauma, she'd disappear. Her eyes would unfocus, her body would go still, and she'd lose the ability to form complete sentences. "I'm fine," she'd say in a voice devoid of inflection, while being anything but fine. Her window was so narrow that any emotional activation immediately triggered shutdown.

Individual Variations in Tolerance Windows

Everyone's window is unique, shaped by genetics, early experiences, trauma history, and learned coping strategies. Some people naturally have wider windows—they're the ones who stay calm in crises, who can tolerate intense emotions without losing themselves. Others have naturally narrower windows, getting overwhelmed more easily. Neither is better or worse—they're just different starting points.

Early attachment profoundly shapes the window of tolerance. Secure attachment, with consistent co-regulation from caregivers, creates a wider, more flexible window. The nervous system learns that stress is manageable, that others will help, that calm will return. But insecure attachment, especially disorganized attachment, creates a narrow, rigid window. The nervous system never learns to trust that regulation is possible.

Cultural factors influence windows too. In cultures where emotional expression is encouraged, people might develop wider tolerance for emotional intensity. In cultures where emotional restraint is valued,

64

the window might be narrower for strong feelings but wider for containing them. There's no universal "healthy" window—context matters.

Current life circumstances affect window width. A supportive relationship can widen your window—you can handle more because you're not alone. Chronic stress narrows it—you're already depleted, so it takes less to push you outside your zone. This is why the same person might have good days where they handle everything smoothly and bad days where tiny things send them into meltdown.

Some people have asymmetric windows. They might tolerate anger well but not sadness, or handle fear but not joy. I had a client who could stay regulated through intense professional challenges but would dissociate at any hint of tenderness. His window was wide for some experiences, narrow for others, shaped by what had been safe and dangerous in his history.

Mapping Edges and Capacity for Regulation

Mapping the edges of someone's window is crucial for effective treatment. We need to know where the edges are, what happens when they're crossed, and what brings someone back inside. This isn't about avoiding the edges—growth happens there—but about knowing where they are so we can work with them skillfully.

I use a simple visual with clients. We draw a rectangle—their window. The top edge is where hyperarousal starts, the bottom where hypoarousal begins. Then we fill in what each zone looks and feels like for them specifically. What are the early warning signs that they're approaching an edge? What are the triggers that push them over? What helps them come back?

For the upper edge, we might note: "First sign: thoughts speed up. Then: jaw clenches, breath gets shallow. If it continues: heart races, hands shake, want to run." For the lower edge: "First sign: feel heavy. Then: hard to follow conversation, vision seems flat. If it continues: can't feel body, words don't make sense, time stops."

Then we map what helps at each stage. Early signs might need just a deep breath or brief movement. Closer to the edge might require stepping outside, splashing cold water on the face, or calling a friend. Once outside the window, different interventions are needed—often opposite ones for hyper versus hypo arousal.

The goal isn't to avoid ever leaving the window—that's impossible and wouldn't lead to growth anyway. The goal is to recognize when you're approaching or crossing an edge, have tools to work with that state, and build capacity to return to the window more quickly. It's about developing flexibility, not rigidity.

We also map patterns. Does the client tend to go up or down when stressed? Do they swing between extremes or get stuck in one zone? Are there predictable sequences—like always going through anger before hitting numbness? These patterns tell us about their nervous system's learned responses and where intervention might be most effective.

The Relationship Between Trauma History and Window Narrowing

Different types of trauma affect the window of tolerance in different ways. Single-incident trauma in adulthood might create specific triggers that push someone outside their window but leave the overall window relatively intact. Complex developmental trauma, on the other hand, often creates a globally narrow window that affects all areas of life.

Early trauma has the most profound effect because the window of tolerance develops alongside the nervous system. If you're experiencing chaos or neglect while your nervous system is still forming, your window develops narrow and rigid. The baseline becomes dysregulation rather than regulation. The window isn't something that got broken—it never got properly built in the first place.

Chronic trauma creates a progressively narrowing window. Each traumatic experience teaches the nervous system that the world is more dangerous than previously thought, so the margins of safety get smaller. People might describe how they used to be able to handle things that now completely overwhelm them. Their window has literally shrunk from repeated threat.

Different trauma types create different window patterns. Sexual trauma often creates a very narrow window around intimacy and touch but might leave other areas relatively intact. Combat trauma might narrow the window around sudden noises and crowds but not affect one-on-one relationships. Emotional abuse might create a narrow window for criticism but not for physical challenges.

The age at which trauma occurred matters enormously. Preverbal trauma—before we have words to make sense of experience—often creates the narrowest windows because the dysregulation gets encoded in the body without cognitive understanding. The nervous system learns that existence itself is threatening, creating a globally narrow window that affects every aspect of life.

Working With Your Window

Understanding your window of tolerance isn't about judgment—it's about awareness. There's nothing wrong with having a narrow window. It's your nervous system's attempt to keep you safe based on what it learned from your experiences. The narrow window that frustrates you now might have literally saved your life during trauma.

But we can work with our windows. They're not fixed. Through consistent experiences of safety, through building regulatory resources, through healing relationships, windows can expand. It's slow work—the nervous system changes gradually, cautiously. But I've seen people whose windows were barely slivers develop the capacity to tolerate and even enjoy a wide range of experiences.

The key is titration—working at the edges without overwhelming the system. If we push too hard, too fast, we retraumatize and the window actually narrows further. But if we never approach the edges, no growth happens. It's like physical exercise—we need just the right amount of challenge to build strength without injury.

This framework also helps us understand why some days are harder than others. Your window isn't static—it breathes, expands and contracts based on countless factors. Instead of beating yourself up for having a "bad day," you can recognize, "My window is narrow today. I need to be gentler with myself, lower the demands, add more support."

Most importantly, understanding windows helps us recognize that everyone—therapists included—has limits to what they can tolerate without dysregulation. This isn't weakness; it's being human. The question isn't whether you have a window of tolerance but how well you know yours and how skillfully you can work with it.

Chapter 9: Clinical Strategies for Window Expansion

The breakthrough came during our fourteenth session. David had been stuck for months, bouncing between panic and numbness with no middle ground. We'd tried everything—breathing exercises, grounding techniques, cognitive restructuring. Nothing stuck. Then one afternoon, as he was describing yet another panic attack, I asked him to slow down. "Just for a moment," I said, "can you feel your feet on the floor?" He paused, looked confused, then surprised. "Yeah, I can. They're... heavy. Solid." For the first time in our work together, he'd found a tiny island of calm within the storm. That was the beginning of expanding his window of tolerance.

Expanding the window of tolerance isn't about eliminating difficult emotions or never feeling overwhelmed again. It's about gradually increasing your capacity to stay present with whatever life throws at you without getting knocked into hyperarousal or collapse. Think of it like strength training for your nervous system—we're building resilience through carefully calibrated challenges, not through overwhelming force.

What makes window expansion so powerful is that it's not just symptom management. When we expand someone's window, we're literally rewiring their nervous system, creating new neural pathways that didn't exist before. Each time someone successfully stays regulated through something that previously would have dysregulated them, they're proving to their nervous system that they can handle more than they thought. It's experiential learning at the deepest level.

Progressive Muscle Relaxation and Guided Imagery Techniques

Progressive muscle relaxation (PMR) works because it speaks directly to the body in a language it understands—tension and release.

When we're chronically stressed or traumatized, our muscles hold patterns of activation or collapse that keep sending danger signals to the brain. PMR interrupts these patterns, teaching the nervous system the difference between tension and relaxation, teaching it that it's safe to let go.

But here's what most people don't realize about PMR with trauma survivors: the traditional approach can actually be triggering. Asking someone to tense their muscles when they're already hypervigilant can push them further into sympathetic activation. Or asking someone in dorsal shutdown to "relax" muscles they can't even feel can increase dissociation. We need to adapt the technique to match where someone's window is right now.

For clients prone to hyperarousal, I use what I call "gentle PMR." Instead of tensing muscles first, we start by simply noticing existing tension. "Can you find a place in your body that feels tight right now? Don't change it, just notice it." Then we imagine that tension slowly melting, like ice cream on a warm day. No force, no effort, just allowing. This avoids adding more activation to an already activated system.

For those stuck in hypoarousal, we need the opposite approach. Here, creating some tension can actually help them feel their body again. But we do it carefully, starting with small movements. "Can you make a fist? Just gently. Now notice what that feels like. Can you make it a tiny bit tighter? Now let it go slowly." We're using the tension to wake up proprioceptors, to bring sensation back online.

Guided imagery takes this further by engaging the imagination to create physiological changes. But again, the images need to match the person's window. Someone hyperaroused doesn't need images of lying on a beach—that much stillness might feel threatening. They might do better imagining themselves walking slowly through a forest, movement with calm. Someone hypoaroused might need images with more energy—a waterfall, sunlight breaking through clouds, spring flowers opening.

I worked with Sandra, a nurse with PTSD from pandemic trauma. Traditional relaxation made her panic—stillness reminded her of patients who'd stopped breathing. So we created imagery of gentle movement: leaves rustling in wind, waves lapping on shore, clouds drifting across sky. Movement that was calm, predictable, safe. Her window began expanding not through forced relaxation but through finding safety in gentle motion.

Titrated Exposure and Pendulation Practices

Titration is the secret sauce of window expansion. Instead of flooding someone with overwhelming experience (which just retraumatizes), we work with tiny, manageable doses. Think of it like homeopathy for the nervous system—just enough challenge to create change without overwhelming the system's capacity to integrate.

The word "pendulation" comes from Peter Levine's Somatic Experiencing, and it describes the natural rhythm of the nervous system—moving between activation and settling, tension and ease. When trauma disrupts this pendulum, we get stuck at the extremes. The practice involves consciously guiding attention between activation and calm, teaching the nervous system to move fluidly between states again.

Here's how it works in practice. Let's say someone gets triggered thinking about their trauma. Instead of diving into the trauma story, we touch it lightly. "When you think about that event, what do you notice in your body?" They might say their chest gets tight. "Okay, can you find somewhere in your body that feels okay, even good?" Maybe their feet feel solid. "Let's just go back and forth. Feel the tight chest for a moment... now the solid feet... back to the chest—is it the same or different?... now the feet again."

What we're doing is teaching the nervous system that activation doesn't have to lead to overwhelm. There's always somewhere else to go, something else to feel. The activation isn't permanent or all-consuming. There's a natural rhythm of expansion and contraction, and we can influence it.

71

Mark came to me unable to drive after a car accident. Even thinking about driving sent him into panic. We started with the tiniest exposure—looking at a picture of his car keys for three seconds, then immediately shifting attention to his breath. Back to the keys for five seconds, then to the feeling of his feet on the ground. Keys for ten seconds, then squeezing a stress ball. We spent three sessions just with the picture before moving to holding actual keys. Six months later, he was driving again. Not because we flooded him with exposure, but because we titrated it so carefully that his window gradually expanded to hold the experience.

Grounding Techniques for Hyperarousal States

When someone's in hyperarousal, they're literally untethered—disconnected from their body, from the present, from the ground beneath them. Grounding techniques work by reestablishing these connections, pulling awareness back from catastrophic futures or traumatic pasts into the manageable present.

The 5-4-3-2-1 technique is popular because it works. Five things you can see, four you can hear, three you can touch, two you can smell, one you can taste. But I've found it works better when we adapt it to the person. Someone with visual trauma might need to skip the seeing part. Someone with eating disorders might struggle with taste. The principle—engaging the senses—matters more than the specific formula.

Physical grounding often works fastest. Holding ice cubes, splashing cold water on the face, doing wall pushups—these create immediate sensory input that's hard to ignore. But the key is finding what works for each person. I had a client who grounded by smelling peppermint oil. Another who carried a smooth stone and rubbed it when activated. Another who did multiplication tables in her head—the cognitive effort pulled her out of emotional overwhelm.

Movement-based grounding can be particularly effective. Stomping feet, shaking hands, bouncing on toes—these discharge the mobilization energy of sympathetic activation while keeping the person present. It's like giving the nervous system something productive to do with all that activation instead of letting it spin into panic.

But here's the thing about grounding—it's not just about calming down in the moment. Each successful grounding experience expands the window slightly. The nervous system learns, "Oh, I can feel this activated and not lose myself. I can bring myself back." Over time, what once required intense grounding techniques might just need a deep breath.

Gentle Activation for Hypoarousal States

Hypoarousal is trickier than hyperarousal because the very circuits we need for activation are offline. Telling someone in dorsal shutdown to "energize" is like telling someone in a coma to wake up—the mechanism for responding isn't available. We need gentle, gradual approaches that coax the nervous system back online without triggering defensive responses.

Temperature is often the gentlest way in. A cool washcloth on the face, holding a cold drink, opening a window for fresh air—these create just enough sensory input to begin mobilization. Heat can work too—a warm compress, hot tea, sunshine through a window. The key is novelty and contrast—something different enough from the numbness to be noticed.

Rhythm and music can penetrate dorsal shutdown when nothing else can. Drumming, even just tapping on knees, creates a rhythm the nervous system can organize around. Music with a strong beat—not necessarily fast, just clear—gives the nervous system something to sync with. I keep a collection of different music styles because what mobilizes one person might further shut down another.

Gentle movement is crucial, but "gentle" is the operative word. We're not trying to activate into sympathetic arousal—we're trying to create just enough mobilization to come back into the window. This might be slowly rolling shoulders, gently stretching arms overhead, or even

73

just wiggling fingers and toes. Start where the person is, not where you think they should be.

Lisa would come to sessions barely able to speak, eyes unfocused, moving like she was underwater. Traditional activation techniques made her panic. So we started with the tiniest movements—blinking deliberately, swallowing consciously, pressing her tongue against the roof of her mouth. These micro-movements began to bring her nervous system back online without triggering defensive responses. From there we could gradually increase—turning her head, lifting her shoulders, eventually standing and stretching.

Somatic Awareness and Interoception Development

Interoception—awareness of internal bodily signals—is often compromised in trauma. People either feel too much (hypervigilance to every sensation) or too little (disconnection from the body). Developing balanced interoception is crucial for window expansion because it's how we know where we are on the arousal spectrum and what we need to regulate.

We start with the most basic sensations. Can you feel your heartbeat? Not count it, just feel it? Can you notice your breathing without changing it? Can you sense whether you're hungry or full, hot or cold, tense or relaxed? For many trauma survivors, these simple questions are surprisingly difficult to answer.

Body scans can develop interoception, but they need to be trauma-informed. Instead of the traditional head-to-toe scan, which can be overwhelming, I use what I call "spotlight scanning." We pick one small area—maybe just the left hand—and spend time really sensing it. Temperature, tension, tingling, numbness, whatever's there. Then we take a break, talk about something else, then maybe scan the right hand. Building tolerance gradually.

The window of tolerance for sensation itself needs expanding. Someone might only be able to tolerate feeling their body for ten seconds before dissociating. So we start with five seconds. Then

74

seven. Then ten. Each increase is an expansion of their window—not just for external stress but for internal experience.

Naming sensations helps integrate them. But we need a vocabulary beyond "good" or "bad." Is it sharp or dull? Moving or still? Hot or cold? Tight or loose? Heavy or light? Spreading or contained? This differentiation helps the nervous system organize sensation rather than being overwhelmed by it.

The Art of Gradual Expansion

Window expansion isn't a linear process. Some days the window will be wider, others narrower. This isn't failure—it's the natural breathing of a living system. What matters is the overall trajectory. Are there more moments of regulation than there were last month? Can they stay present with experiences that used to trigger immediate dysregulation?

The key is working at the edge of the window without going over. Too little challenge and no growth happens. Too much and we retraumatize, potentially narrowing the window further. It's like physical therapy after an injury—we need just the right amount of stretch to promote healing without reinjuring.

Each person's window expansion will look different. For one person, being able to sit through a full therapy session without dissociating is huge progress. For another, it might be handling criticism without rage. For another, feeling sadness without collapse. We're not aiming for some universal standard of regulation—we're helping each person expand their unique capacity.

Most importantly, window expansion is about more than just tolerating more stress. It's about increasing our capacity for joy, connection, creativity, play—all the experiences that require us to stay present and engaged. As the window expands, life itself expands. Things that were impossible become possible. The world literally becomes a bigger, richer place.

The techniques I've shared are tools, not rules. Use them flexibly, creatively, always in service of the person in front of you. And remember—every small expansion matters. Every moment someone stays regulated through something that used to dysregulate them is a victory. These victories accumulate, building resilience one experience at a time.

Chapter 10: Building Resilience and Autonomic Flexibility

My client Rebecca sat across from me, frustrated. "I do everything right," she said. "Therapy twice a week, meditation every morning, yoga every evening. But I still fall apart when my boss raises his voice. What am I doing wrong?" She wasn't doing anything wrong. She was learning what we all need to understand: resilience isn't about never getting dysregulated. It's about how quickly you can find your way back to center when life knocks you off balance.

Autonomic flexibility—the ability to move appropriately between different nervous system states based on actual circumstances—is the hallmark of a healthy nervous system. It's not about being calm all the time. Sometimes we need sympathetic activation to meet a deadline or handle an emergency. Sometimes we need dorsal withdrawal to rest and restore. The problem isn't having these states; it's getting stuck in them.

Building resilience is like creating a robust ecosystem in your nervous system. A single tree might fall in a storm, but a forest with diverse trees, underground root networks, and multiple layers of vegetation can weather almost anything. We're not trying to become invulnerable. We're building multiple pathways back to regulation, so when one path gets blocked, we have others.

Mindfulness and Self-Compassion Practices

Mindfulness often gets misunderstood as being about emptying your mind or feeling peaceful all the time. But mindfulness for trauma survivors is different. It's about developing dual awareness—the ability to notice what's happening in your nervous system while simultaneously remembering that you're the one noticing. This observer perspective is what keeps us from drowning in our experience.

The problem with traditional mindfulness for trauma survivors is that turning attention inward can be triggering. Sitting still, closing eyes, focusing on breath—for someone whose trauma involved immobilization, this can trigger massive defensive responses. So we need trauma-informed mindfulness that respects the nervous system's needs for safety.

I teach what I call "anchored mindfulness." Instead of free-floating awareness that can drift into dissociation or overwhelm, we always keep one foot in external reality. Eyes open or easily opened. Awareness of the room, sounds, temperature. Then from this anchored place, we can safely notice internal experience. "I'm sitting in this chair, in this room, and I notice my heart is racing." The external anchor keeps us from getting lost.

Self-compassion is equally crucial for resilience, but it's often the hardest thing for trauma survivors to develop. Their nervous systems learned that self-criticism might keep them safer—if they could figure out what they did wrong, maybe they could prevent future harm. But this internal criticism actually narrows the window of tolerance by adding threat from the inside.

Kristin Neff's three components of self-compassion—kindness, common humanity, and mindfulness—map beautifully onto nervous system regulation. Kindness activates the ventral vagal care system. Common humanity reminds us we're not alone, supporting co-regulation even when alone. Mindfulness keeps us present rather than lost in rumination or dissociation.

But we can't just tell someone to be self-compassionate. For many, the very attempt triggers shame or anger. So we start small. Can you be 1% less critical? Can you talk to yourself like you'd talk to a good friend in the same situation? Can you put your hand on your heart when you're struggling, even if you don't feel compassionate? These small gestures begin to rewire the nervous system toward self-soothing rather than self-attack.

Interpersonal Effectiveness Training

Relationships are where our nervous systems learn regulation or dysregulation, and they're also where healing happens. But for trauma survivors, relationships can feel like minefields. Every interaction carries the potential for triggering old wounds. Building interpersonal effectiveness means learning to navigate relationships while maintaining nervous system regulation.

Boundaries are crucial for autonomic flexibility. Without boundaries, we're constantly at the mercy of others' states—their anxiety becomes our anxiety, their anger triggers our defenses. But rigid boundaries cut us off from the co-regulation we need. Healthy boundaries are semipermeable—they let in what nourishes and keep out what harms.

Teaching boundaries through a nervous system lens changes everything. Instead of rules about what's acceptable, we learn to notice body signals. That tightness in your chest when someone stands too close? That's your nervous system saying "boundary needed." That warmth when someone respects your no? That's your nervous system saying "safety confirmed." The body becomes our boundary guide.

Communication skills matter, but they have to work when we're dysregulated, not just when we're calm. I teach what I call "state-aware communication." First, recognize what state you're in. If you're in sympathetic activation, you might need to say, "I need five minutes before we talk." If you're in dorsal shutdown, you might text instead of calling. Matching communication to your nervous system state prevents relationships from becoming dysregulating.

Conflict resolution through a Polyvagal lens focuses on maintaining co-regulation even during disagreement. This doesn't mean avoiding conflict—that's often impossible and unhealthy. It means recognizing when one or both people have left their window of tolerance and pausing to regulate before continuing. "I can feel myself getting activated. Can we take a break and come back to this?" This isn't avoidance; it's wisdom.

Physical Practices: Yoga, Martial Arts, and Movement Therapies

Movement is medicine for the nervous system, but not all movement is created equal. The right kind of movement can expand the window of tolerance, build resilience, and create new patterns of regulation. The wrong kind can retraumatize or reinforce dysregulation patterns.

Yoga has become almost synonymous with trauma healing, and for good reason. The combination of breath, movement, and awareness speaks directly to the nervous system. But trauma-sensitive yoga is different from regular yoga. We never force poses, we always offer choices, and we focus on internal experience rather than external form. It's not about touching your toes; it's about noticing what happens in your nervous system as you move.

Different yoga practices affect the nervous system differently. Vigorous flow can help discharge sympathetic activation—great for someone stuck in anxiety or anger. Gentle, supported poses can help mobilize from dorsal shutdown. Restorative yoga can teach the nervous system that stillness can be safe. The key is matching the practice to the person's window and gradually expanding from there.

Martial arts offer something unique—the integration of power and control. For trauma survivors who felt powerless, learning to strike, block, and move with intention can be profoundly healing. But it's not about becoming aggressive. It's about knowing you have power and choosing when and how to use it. This builds a different kind of confidence—embodied confidence that changes how you move through the world.

Dance and expressive movement work with the nervous system's natural rhythms. Unlike structured exercise, expressive movement lets the body move how it needs to move. Shaking, swaying, stomping—these aren't just emotional expressions; they're nervous system regulation strategies. Animals shake after trauma to discharge the energy. Humans have socialized ourselves out of this natural response, but we can reclaim it.

I worked with James, a veteran who couldn't sit still in therapy. Talking made him more agitated. So we started walking during sessions, then eventually joined a boxing gym together. As he learned to channel his activation through controlled movement, his window expanded. The ring became a place where sympathetic activation was appropriate, even useful. This gave his nervous system permission to activate without shame and, paradoxically, made it easier to downregulate afterward.

Self-Care Routines and Lifestyle Factors

Self-care isn't selfish—it's nervous system maintenance. Just like a car needs regular oil changes, our nervous system needs regular care to function well. But self-care for trauma survivors isn't just bubble baths and face masks. It's about creating routines that support nervous system regulation throughout the day.

Sleep is fundamental. A dysregulated nervous system disrupts sleep, and poor sleep further dysregulates the nervous system. It's a vicious cycle. But instead of perfect sleep hygiene (which can become its own source of stress), we focus on creating safety for sleep. This might mean nightlights for someone whose trauma happened in the dark, or white noise for someone who needs to mask triggering sounds.

Nutrition affects the nervous system more than most people realize. Blood sugar swings can trigger sympathetic activation. Dehydration can trigger dorsal shutdown. Caffeine can narrow the window of tolerance. But instead of strict diets, we focus on nervous system-friendly eating: regular meals, adequate protein, enough water. Notice how different foods affect your state. Some people find sugar dysregulating; others find it soothing. There's no universal prescription.

Daily rhythms create predictability that supports regulation. This doesn't mean rigid schedules but reliable patterns. Morning routines that transition from sleep to waking. Evening routines that signal the nervous system to downregulate. Regular meal times that prevent blood sugar crashes. These rhythms become external regulators for an internal system that struggles to self-regulate.

Social rhythms matter too. Regular connection with safe others. Predictable alone time for introverts. Balance between stimulation and rest. The pandemic taught us how much our nervous systems rely on these social rhythms. Without them, even resilient people struggled with regulation.

Creating Personalized Regulation Toolkits

One size doesn't fit all when it comes to nervous system regulation. What soothes one person might activate another. What energizes one might exhaust another. That's why everyone needs their own personalized toolkit—a collection of strategies that work for their unique nervous system.

The toolkit needs different tools for different states. For sympathetic activation: What helps you discharge energy? What helps you slow down? What reminds you you're safe? For dorsal shutdown: What gently mobilizes you? What helps you feel your body? What connects you to the present? For the window of tolerance: What keeps you centered? What prevents dysregulation? What supports flexibility?

But here's the crucial part—the toolkit needs to be accessible when you're dysregulated. Complex breathing exercises might be great when you're calm but impossible when you're panicking. So we need simple, body-based tools that work even when thinking is offline. A smooth stone in your pocket. A photo on your phone. A playlist ready to go. A friend you can text.

I encourage clients to create actual physical toolkits. A box or bag with tangible items: essential oils for scent, stress balls for touch, photos for vision, playlists for sound, mints for taste. When dysregulated, you don't have to think—just reach for the box. The act of choosing a tool is itself regulating.

Digital toolkits matter too. Apps that guide breathing. Playlists organized by state—one for calming, one for energizing, one for focusing. Photos organized by effect—ones that make you smile, ones that remind you of your strength, ones that connect you to loved ones. Voice memos from your regulated self to your dysregulated self.

The toolkit grows over time. Something that works in early recovery might not work later. Something that never worked before might suddenly click. The toolkit isn't fixed—it's a living collection that changes as you change. And sharing toolkits with others can be powerful. What works for someone else might work for you, or might inspire you to try something new.

Building Your Resilient Life

Resilience isn't about becoming bulletproof. It's about becoming flexible, adaptable, responsive rather than reactive. It's about having multiple strategies for returning to regulation, multiple sources of support, multiple ways of being in the world. It's about trusting your nervous system's capacity to handle challenge and return to balance.

Building resilience takes time. The nervous system changes slowly, cautiously. It needs repeated experiences of successfully handling stress and returning to calm. It needs evidence that the new patterns are reliable, that safety is possible, that connection won't lead to harm. Be patient with yourself. You're not just changing habits; you're rewiring neural pathways laid down over a lifetime.

The practices I've described aren't prescriptions—they're possibilities. Try things. Notice what helps. Keep what works, leave what doesn't. Your nervous system is your guide. It knows what it needs, even if that knowing isn't yet conscious. Trust the wisdom of your body, even as you gently encourage it toward new patterns.

And remember, resilience isn't an individual achievement. We're social creatures, designed to regulate in relationship. Building resilience means building connections, finding your people, creating networks of support. It means both learning to self-regulate and allowing co-regulation. It means being both strong and vulnerable, independent and interdependent.

The goal isn't to never need support or never feel overwhelmed. The goal is to develop enough flexibility that you can navigate whatever life brings—sometimes with grace, sometimes messily, but always with the knowledge that you can find your way back to center. That's true resilience.

Chapter 11: Polyvagal-Informed EMDR Fundamentals

The first time I tried to use EMDR with a client in dorsal shutdown, it was a disaster. Sarah sat there, eyes glazed, mechanically following the bilateral stimulation while clearly not present at all. We were going through the motions, but nothing was happening. Her nervous system wasn't available for processing—it had checked out to protect her. That's when I realized EMDR without understanding autonomic states is like trying to start a car without checking if there's gas in the tank.

When Francine Shapiro discovered EMDR in the late 1980s, she gave us a powerful tool for trauma processing. But when we combine EMDR with Polyvagal Theory, something magical happens. We stop just following protocols and start working with the actual biological state of the person in front of us. We can see when someone's nervous system is ready for processing and when it needs more preparation. We understand why some people get flooded during bilateral stimulation while others dissociate.

The integration of these two approaches isn't just theoretical—it's intensely practical. Every phase of EMDR can be enhanced by understanding what's happening in the autonomic nervous system. Every stuck point in processing makes more sense when viewed through a Polyvagal lens. And most importantly, we can make EMDR safer and more effective by ensuring the nervous system is actually available for the work we're asking it to do.

The Synergy Between Adaptive Information Processing and Polyvagal Theory

Shapiro's Adaptive Information Processing (AIP) model tells us that trauma gets stuck because overwhelming experiences don't get properly processed and stored. The memory networks remain frozen in time, with all the original emotions, body sensations, and beliefs intact. When triggered, these networks activate as if the trauma is happening now. Sound familiar? That's exactly what Polyvagal Theory describes—a nervous system stuck in defensive responses to past threats.

According to research by van der Kolk and colleagues, traumatic memories are stored differently than normal memories. They're fragmented, sensory-based, and disconnected from our usual narrative memory system. From a Polyvagal perspective, this makes perfect sense. When we're in sympathetic activation or dorsal shutdown, the parts of our brain responsible for coherent narrative processing go offline. The memory gets encoded in the state it was experienced—chaos or collapse.

The beauty of combining these models is that we can understand not just what needs to happen (processing stuck memories) but what needs to be present for it to happen (sufficient nervous system regulation). The AIP model tells us the memories need to link up with adaptive information. Polyvagal Theory tells us this linking can only happen when we're in our window of tolerance, with access to our ventral vagal state.

Think about it—when you're in fight-or-flight, you're not making new connections or seeing things from different perspectives. You're just trying to survive. The same is true during EMDR. If someone's nervous system is in defensive mode, they can't access the adaptive perspectives and resources needed for processing. They're just reliving the trauma, not transforming it.

This explains why some people seem to "resist" EMDR or why processing gets stuck. It's not resistance—it's nervous system protection. Their autonomic state is saying, "This is too dangerous to process right now." Instead of pushing through (which can be retraumatizing), we need to work with the nervous system, building safety and capacity first.

How Memory Storage Relates to Autonomic States

Research by Ogden and colleagues shows that traumatic memories are stored with the autonomic state that was active during the trauma. If you were in sympathetic hyperarousal during the event, the memory includes that activation. If you dissociated into dorsal shutdown, that's part of the memory too. This is why triggering a trauma memory often triggers the same autonomic state—the whole package gets activated together.

During EMDR, we're asking people to activate these state-dependent memories while maintaining dual attention—one foot in the past, one in the present. But here's the thing: if the stored autonomic state is too intense, it overwhelms the person's current regulation capacity. They lose dual attention and fall completely into the trauma state. The bilateral stimulation isn't resourcing—it's retraumatizing.

This is where Polyvagal awareness changes everything. By tracking autonomic states during processing, we can titrate the work. If someone starts shifting toward the edge of their window, we can pause, resource, and regulate before continuing. We're not just watching for cognitive or emotional overwhelm—we're tracking the biological capacity to stay present.

I worked with Marcus, a firefighter with PTSD from a fatal fire. Every time we targeted the memory, his sympathetic system would explode—heart racing, sweating, muscles tensing for action. His body was preparing to run into that burning building again. We had to work first on expanding his window of tolerance, teaching his nervous system that he could feel activation without losing himself in it. Only then could EMDR be effective.

Different autonomic states also affect what information is accessible during processing. In ventral vagal, people can access compassion, perspective, and connection. In sympathetic, they might access anger or fear but not self-compassion. In dorsal, they might feel nothing at all. Understanding this helps us know what's possible in each moment of processing.

Neuro-Informed History Taking Through a Polyvagal Lens

Traditional EMDR history-taking focuses on trauma events, symptoms, and negative beliefs. Polyvagal-informed history-taking adds another layer—mapping the client's autonomic patterns. We're not just asking what happened; we're asking what happened to their nervous system and how it adapted.

Research by Corrigan and colleagues emphasizes the importance of understanding not just trauma content but trauma impact on the nervous system. When taking history, I ask questions like: "When that happened, did you fight back, run away, or freeze?" "Did you feel like you left your body?" "Was there a moment when you just gave up?" These questions help identify which autonomic states were active during trauma and might be stored with the memory.

We also explore current autonomic patterns. "What happens in your body when you think about the trauma?" "Do you tend to get anxious or numb?" "What helps you feel calm and present?" This gives us a map of their current nervous system functioning—where they get stuck, what resources they have, and what we need to build before processing.

The history includes identifying triggers and glimmers specific to their nervous system. What shifts them into defense? What brings them back to safety? This informs our preparation phase—which resources will actually work for this particular nervous system—and our processing phase—which memories might be too activating to start with.

I also assess for developmental trauma's impact on the nervous system. Early trauma often creates globally narrow windows of tolerance and limited access to ventral vagal states. These clients need extensive preparation before EMDR. Their nervous systems literally don't have the infrastructure for standard processing. We have to build it first.

Optimizing Biological Responses Throughout the Eight Phases

Each of EMDR's eight phases can be enhanced by incorporating Polyvagal awareness. In Phase 1 (History), we're mapping both trauma history and autonomic patterns. In Phase 2 (Preparation), we're explicitly building nervous system regulation capacity, not just cognitive resources.

According to research by Siegel and Solomon, the preparation phase is crucial for EMDR success. From a Polyvagal perspective, this phase is about expanding the window of tolerance and building ventral vagal capacity. We're teaching the nervous system that it can handle activation without overwhelm, that it can touch trauma and return to safety.

Phase 3 (Assessment) involves activating the trauma memory network. Here, we need to ensure the person has enough regulation to maintain dual attention. If activating the memory sends them outside their window, we need to back up and do more preparation. The target isn't ready if the nervous system isn't ready.

Phases 4-6 (Desensitization, Installation, Body Scan) require careful state monitoring. Is the bilateral stimulation regulating or dysregulating? Are they processing or just surviving? I watch for signs of state shifts—changes in breathing, posture, eye contact—and adjust accordingly. Sometimes we need to slow down, sometimes shift to less activating bilateral stimulation, sometimes pause to resource.

Phase 7 (Closure) is about ensuring the nervous system is regulated before ending. This isn't just checking if they're cognitively okay—it's ensuring their autonomic state is settled. We might need extended closure with regulation exercises, grounding, or co-regulation to help them leave in a ventral vagal state.

Phase 8 (Reevaluation) includes checking not just if the memory is still disturbing but how their nervous system responds to it. Has their window of tolerance expanded? Can they think about the trauma without state shifts? This tells us if the processing is truly complete or if the nervous system still holds protective responses.

Maintaining Dual Attention Through Co-Regulation

Dual attention—keeping awareness of present safety while processing past trauma—is essential for EMDR. But maintaining dual attention requires sufficient nervous system regulation. When someone's in sympathetic overload or dorsal collapse, dual attention becomes impossible. They're either all in the past or completely disconnected.

This is where therapist co-regulation becomes crucial. According to research by Schore on right-brain to right-brain communication in therapy, our regulated nervous system can help stabilize our client's nervous system during processing. Our calm presence, steady voice, and regulated breathing provide an anchor to the present.

During bilateral stimulation, I'm constantly offering co-regulatory cues. My voice stays steady and grounded. I might say, "Notice my voice... you're here with me... that was then, this is now." These aren't just cognitive reminders—they're nervous system anchors. My regulated state helps their nervous system remember safety exists.

Sometimes co-regulation means adjusting our physical presence. Moving slightly closer if someone's dissociating, creating more space if they're activated. Modulating our voice—softer for hyperarousal, more energized for hypoarousal. We're using our nervous system as a tuning fork to help theirs find regulation.

I learned this with Amy, who would dissociate every time we processed her abuse memories. Standard grounding techniques didn't work—she was too far gone. What worked was me gently humming

90

while doing bilateral stimulation. The vibration of humming, combined with bilateral stimulation, kept just enough activation to prevent complete shutdown while the consistent rhythm provided safety. Her nervous system could borrow my regulation to stay present enough for processing.

The Integration That Changes Everything

When we bring Polyvagal Theory into EMDR, we're not just adding another technique—we're fundamentally changing how we understand and facilitate healing. We're working with the wisdom of the body, respecting the protective intelligence of the nervous system, and creating conditions for natural processing to occur.

This integration helps explain EMDR phenomena that were mysterious before. Why does bilateral stimulation work? Perhaps because it mimics the natural oscillation of a regulated nervous system. Why do some people process quickly while others take months of preparation? Because their nervous systems have different levels of regulation and resilience.

Most importantly, this integration makes EMDR more attuned and safer. We're not pushing through defensive responses—we're working with them. We're not overwhelming already overwhelmed nervous systems—we're building capacity first. We're not just processing memories—we're helping nervous systems learn they can touch trauma and return to safety.

The combination of AIP and Polyvagal Theory gives us a complete picture. AIP shows us what needs to happen—stuck memories need to connect with adaptive information. Polyvagal Theory shows us what needs to be present for it to happen—sufficient nervous system regulation and window of tolerance. Together, they create a framework for truly holistic trauma treatment.

As you integrate these approaches, trust the wisdom of the nervous system. If processing isn't working, check the autonomic state. If someone can't maintain dual attention, build more regulation first. If bilateral stimulation is overwhelming, adjust it to match their window. The nervous system knows what it needs—our job is to listen and respond appropriately.

Chapter 12: Phase-Specific Polyvagal Applications in EMDR

Tom sat in my office, eager to process his combat trauma. He'd done the preparation exercises, learned the safe place visualization, could do butterfly hugs in his sleep. By all standard EMDR measures, he was ready. But when I looked at him through a Polyvagal lens, I saw something different—chronic sympathetic activation masked as readiness. His enthusiasm was actually hypervigilance. His compliance was survival mode. His nervous system wasn't ready; it was braced for impact.

This is why we need phase-specific Polyvagal applications in EMDR. Each phase demands different things from the nervous system, and each phase offers opportunities to build regulation and resilience. When we understand what autonomic state each phase requires and supports, we can work more precisely, more safely, and more effectively.

What I've learned through years of integration is that EMDR phases aren't just procedural steps—they're nervous system experiences. Phase 1 isn't just gathering history; it's establishing safety in the therapeutic relationship. Phase 4 isn't just desensitization; it's teaching the nervous system it can feel activation and return to calm. Every phase becomes an opportunity for nervous system healing when we understand the biology beneath the protocol.

The Preparation Hierarchy Model: Assessing Readiness for Reprocessing

The Preparation Hierarchy Model, developed through clinical observation and supported by research from Korn and Leeds on resource development, recognizes that not everyone needs the same level of preparation. But through a Polyvagal lens, we can be even more precise about what preparation each nervous system needs.

Level 1 preparation is for clients with good nervous system regulation—they have wide windows of tolerance, can move flexibly between states, and have reliable return to baseline. These folks might need just basic safe place and resource installation. Their nervous systems already know how to regulate; we're just adding some EMDR-specific tools.

Level 2 is for moderate dysregulation—narrower windows, some stuck points, but basic capacity for regulation. Here we need to build more resources. According to research by Jarero and colleagues on group treatment protocols, these clients benefit from extended stabilization work. We're teaching breathing techniques, grounding skills, and bilateral stimulation for regulation. We're expanding their window before we start processing.

Level 3 is for severe dysregulation—very narrow windows, limited ventral vagal access, quick shifts to defense. These clients need extensive preparation, sometimes months of building basic regulation capacity. We're not just installing resources; we're literally building the neural pathways for regulation that might never have properly developed.

But here's what standard models miss: readiness isn't static. Someone might be Level 1 for some memories and Level 3 for others. Their nervous system might be ready to process a car accident but not childhood abuse. Or they might be ready on Tuesday but not Thursday, depending on life stressors, sleep, nutrition, and countless other factors affecting their window of tolerance.

I use a simple nervous system check-in to assess readiness each session. Can they feel their feet on the floor? Can they make eye contact without overwhelm? Can they think about the target memory without immediate state shift? If the answer to any of these is no, we need more preparation, regardless of how many resources they've installed.

Phases 1-2: Building Safety and Resources Through Ventral Vagal Activation

Phase 1 (History) through a Polyvagal lens isn't just information gathering—it's co-regulation and safety building. How we take history matters as much as what we learn. Speaking slowly, maintaining warm eye contact, allowing silence—these create ventral vagal conditions that help clients feel safe enough to share.

Research by Fisher on structural dissociation shows that traumatized individuals often have parts of themselves stuck in different autonomic states. During history-taking, we might be talking to a relatively regulated adult part while trauma-holding parts are in sympathetic or dorsal states. We need to acknowledge and work with all parts of their nervous system.

I structure history-taking to avoid overwhelming the nervous system. Instead of diving into trauma details, we start with strengths and resources. What's working in their life? What helps them feel calm? This activates ventral vagal states and builds our co-regulatory connection before we approach difficult material.

Phase 2 (Preparation) is explicitly about building ventral vagal capacity. The classic "safe place" exercise isn't just visualization—it's nervous system programming. When someone imagines their safe place while in a ventral vagal state, then adds bilateral stimulation, they're literally strengthening neural pathways for accessing safety.

But many trauma survivors can't access a safe place because their nervous systems have never known true safety. For them, we might start with "calm place" or even just "okay place." Or we might build resources around activities rather than places—the feeling of petting their dog, listening to music, cooking a familiar meal. Whatever brings even a moment of ventral vagal activation becomes a resource.

Resource installation through bilateral stimulation is more effective when we understand autonomic states. According to research by

Hofmann and colleagues on memory consolidation, positive resources are better integrated when installed during optimal arousal states. Too much activation and the resource won't stick. Too little and there's not enough neuroplasticity. We need that ventral vagal sweet spot.

Phases 3-6: Maintaining Regulation During Reprocessing

Phase 3 (Assessment) requires careful calibration. We're activating the trauma network enough to access it but not so much that we overwhelm the system. From a Polyvagal perspective, we're bringing someone to the edge of their window without pushing them over.

I watch for autonomic shifts as we identify the target. If someone goes into immediate sympathetic activation just naming the memory, we might need to "sneak up" on it. Start with a related but less activating aspect. If someone dissociates when identifying emotions, we might start with body sensations instead. We're titrating activation to match their window.

Phase 4 (Desensitization) is where Polyvagal awareness becomes absolutely critical. Research by van der Kolk and colleagues shows that trauma processing requires the prefrontal cortex to stay online enough to integrate experience. But sympathetic overactivation or dorsal shutdown takes the prefrontal cortex offline. We need to maintain that optimal zone.

During bilateral stimulation, I'm constantly tracking autonomic state. Breathing changes? Posture shifts? Face flushing or paling? These tell me more than SUDs scores about what's happening in their nervous system. If I see signs of moving outside the window, we might slow the bilateral stimulation, shorten sets, or pause to resource.

Different types of bilateral stimulation affect the nervous system differently. Eye movements can be activating for some, regulating for others. Taps might feel soothing or triggering depending on trauma history. Sounds might regulate unless there was auditory trauma. We need to match the bilateral stimulation to what this particular nervous system needs.

Phase 5 (Installation) works better when we understand that positive beliefs can only be integrated in ventral vagal states. If someone's still activated or shut down from processing, the positive belief won't integrate properly. We might need to regulate first, then install. This is why some installations don't "stick"—the nervous system wasn't in a state to receive them.

Phase 6 (Body Scan) is essentially an interoception exercise. But trauma often disrupts interoception. According to research by Payne and colleagues on somatic experiencing, many trauma survivors can't accurately sense their bodies. They might report "nothing" when actually holding significant tension, or "fine" when actually dissociated.

Phase 7-8: Body Scan and Future Template Through Autonomic Awareness

The body scan isn't just checking for remaining activation—it's teaching the nervous system to notice and respond to its own signals. We're building interoceptive awareness, which research by Craig shows is fundamental to emotional regulation and self-awareness.

When someone reports tension during the body scan, we need to differentiate between processing continuation and nervous system dysregulation. Is this the trauma still processing, or is this their nervous system saying "too much"? The quality of the sensation often tells us—processing sensations tend to move and change, while overwhelm sensations tend to be stuck or increasing.

Phase 7 (Closure) requires ensuring not just cognitive closure but autonomic regulation. According to research by Lanius and colleagues on neurobiology of PTSD, traumatized individuals often have delayed emotional reactions. Someone might seem fine at session end but have extreme activation hours later. We need to close in a way that supports continued regulation.

97

I teach clients specific closure practices based on their nervous system patterns. Someone prone to sympathetic activation might need vigorous movement to discharge energy. Someone prone to dorsal shutdown might need gentle activation to stay present. Everyone gets a "regulation plan" for the hours after session.

Phase 8 (Reevaluation) looks different through a Polyvagal lens. We're not just checking if the memory still disturbs them—we're assessing how their nervous system responds. Can they think about it without state shift? Has their window expanded? Are they accessing different autonomic states than before?

Future templating requires ventral vagal access because imagining positive futures requires the social engagement system. If someone can't imagine handling future challenges successfully, it might not be resistance or negative beliefs—their nervous system might literally not have access to those possibilities from its current state.

Managing Abreactions and Dissociation with Polyvagal Interventions

Abreactions—intense emotional and physical reactions during processing—make sense from a Polyvagal perspective. The nervous system is literally re-experiencing the autonomic state from the trauma. According to research by Nijenhuis on somatoform dissociation, these aren't just emotional releases but full-body nervous system responses.

When abreaction happens, standard EMDR says keep going if there's dual attention. But Polyvagal awareness adds nuance. Is this sympathetic discharge that needs to complete, or is this retraumatization? The quality of the experience tells us. Healthy discharge has movement and rhythm. Retraumatization has that stuck, looping quality.

For sympathetic abreactions, I might encourage the discharge while maintaining co-regulation. "Let your body shake... I'm right here... that energy needs to move through." We're supporting the natural completion of the fight-or-flight response that got interrupted during trauma.

Dissociation during EMDR is the nervous system saying "this is too much." But there are different types of dissociation. Research by van der Hart and colleagues on structural dissociation distinguishes between detachment (spacing out) and compartmentalization (parts taking over). Each needs different intervention.

For spacing out dissociation, we need gentle sensory grounding. Change the bilateral stimulation to something more activating. Use voice to anchor. Maybe pause processing and do some movement. We're bringing just enough activation to counter the shutdown without triggering sympathetic overload.

For parts-based dissociation, we might need to work with the part that's emerged. "I notice something shifted. Can you help me understand what's happening?" Often a protective part has activated because the processing touched something too vulnerable. We need to acknowledge and work with the protection, not push through it.

Precision and Compassion in Integration

Integrating Polyvagal Theory with EMDR isn't about making treatment more complicated—it's about making it more precise and compassionate. We're not just following protocols; we're responding to the actual biological state of the person in front of us. Every intervention becomes more targeted when we understand which autonomic state we're working with.

This integration also helps us understand why EMDR works differently for different people. Someone with good nervous system regulation might process trauma in a few sessions. Someone with developmental trauma might need months of preparation just to build enough regulation for processing. Neither is doing it wrong—their nervous systems have different starting points and needs.

Most importantly, this approach reduces retraumatization. By respecting nervous system limits, titrating activation, and ensuring adequate regulation, we make EMDR safer. We're not overwhelming already overwhelmed systems. We're building capacity gradually, teaching the nervous system it can handle what once overwhelmed it.

As you integrate these approaches in your practice, trust what you see more than what protocols say. If someone's nervous system is saying "not ready," believe it, regardless of how many resources they've installed. If bilateral stimulation is dysregulating, adjust it, even if it's "supposed" to work. The nervous system's wisdom supersedes any protocol.

The beautiful thing about combining EMDR with Polyvagal Theory is that we're working with two systems that fundamentally trust the body's ability to heal. EMDR trusts the brain's natural processing ability. Polyvagal Theory trusts the nervous system's protective wisdom. Together, they create a framework for healing that honors both the trauma and the intelligence of our biological responses to it.

Chapter 13: Polyvagal Theory Meets Parts Work

The first time I witnessed the connection between parts and nervous system states, it changed everything about how I practice therapy. My client Jessica was describing her inner critic—that harsh voice that constantly told her she wasn't good enough. "When it shows up," she said, "my whole body changes. I get tense, my breathing gets shallow, I want to disappear." She was describing a part, but she was also describing a nervous system shift from ventral vagal safety into sympathetic activation and then dorsal collapse. That's when it hit me: our parts don't just have different voices and roles—they live in different autonomic states.

Internal Family Systems, developed by Richard Schwartz, teaches us that we all have multiple parts or sub-personalities, each with its own perspective, emotions, and role in our internal system. What happens when we look at these parts through a Polyvagal lens? We discover that each part not only has its own story but its own nervous system state. Some parts keep us in constant sympathetic vigilance. Others pull us into dorsal shutdown. And the Self—that core, compassionate awareness—correlates beautifully with ventral vagal activation.

This integration isn't just theoretically interesting—it's clinically revolutionary. When we understand that parts are organized around autonomic states, we can work with them more precisely. We're not just talking to parts; we're working with the nervous system states they inhabit and protect. This makes the work safer, more effective, and more compassionate for everyone involved—all the parts and the Self that holds them.

Understanding Parts Through Autonomic States

According to research by Schwartz and Sweezy on the IFS model, our parts develop to protect us from overwhelming experiences. But through a Polyvagal lens, we can see that these parts don't just protect us psychologically—they protect us by managing our autonomic states. A part that keeps us angry might be maintaining sympathetic activation to avoid the vulnerability of ventral vagal connection. A part that makes us dissociate might be using dorsal shutdown to escape overwhelming activation.

Think about it this way: every part learned its protective strategy during a specific autonomic state and continues to operate from that state. The part that formed when you were a terrified five-year-old still carries the sympathetic activation of that moment. The part that emerged when you gave up hope still holds the dorsal collapse of that despair. These aren't just psychological patterns—they're embodied nervous system states frozen in time.

I worked with Michael, who had a part that he called "the sergeant"—always scanning for danger, never letting him relax. When we explored this part through a Polyvagal lens, we discovered it lived in permanent sympathetic activation. It literally didn't know any other state existed. It had been protecting Michael since his chaotic childhood by maintaining hypervigilance, and it couldn't imagine safety without that activation.

Different types of parts tend to inhabit different autonomic states. Manager parts—those that try to control and prevent pain—often operate from sympathetic mobilization. They're actively doing, planning, controlling. Firefighter parts—those that react when pain breaks through—might use either extreme sympathetic (rage, panic) or dorsal (dissociation, numbing) strategies. Exiled parts—those that hold the original pain—are often stuck in the autonomic state of the original trauma.

Understanding this helps explain why some parts are so hard to access or work with. A part in deep dorsal shutdown might literally not have the biological activation needed to engage in therapy. A part in extreme sympathetic arousal might not have access to the reflection and perspective-taking that requires ventral vagal activation. We're not just dealing with resistance—we're dealing with biological states that limit what's possible.

Self Energy as Ventral Vagal Activation

Here's where things get really interesting. In IFS, Self is described as our core essence—curious, compassionate, calm, connected. According to research by Schwartz on the nature of Self in IFS, when we're in Self-energy, we naturally embody what he calls the 8 C's: curiosity, compassion, clarity, creativity, calm, confidence, courage, and connectedness. Now look at that list through a Polyvagal lens. Every one of those qualities requires ventral vagal activation.

You literally cannot be genuinely curious when you're in sympathetic fight-or-flight—you're too focused on threat. You cannot access compassion from dorsal shutdown—you're too disconnected. The 8 C's aren't just psychological qualities; they're markers of a regulated nervous system with access to the social engagement system. Self-energy IS ventral vagal activation.

This explains why it's so hard to access Self when we're triggered. It's not just that our parts are louder or more active—it's that the autonomic state required for Self-energy isn't biologically available. When we're in defensive states, the neural circuits for the 8 C's are literally offline. We need a certain level of nervous system regulation to access Self.

I see this clearly with clients. When Sarah arrives activated, speaking rapidly about her week's disasters, she has no access to Self. But as we work together to regulate her nervous system—

through breathing, grounding, co-regulation—suddenly Self emerges. Her voice changes, her perspective shifts, she can hold complexity. She didn't find Self through thinking; she found it through shifting her autonomic state.

This also explains why some traditional IFS techniques might not work for highly dysregulated clients. Asking someone to "go inside and find Self" when their nervous system is in chaos is like asking them to find something in a dark room while the building is on fire. We need to help regulate the nervous system first, creating the biological conditions for Self to emerge.

Mapping Parts on the Autonomic Hierarchy

When we map parts onto the autonomic hierarchy, patterns emerge that help both therapist and client understand the internal system better. According to research by Dana on clinical applications of Polyvagal Theory, creating visual maps helps clients understand their nervous system patterns. The same is true for parts—when we map them onto the autonomic ladder, the whole system becomes clearer.

At the top of the ladder, in ventral vagal, we find Self and any parts that have been unburdened and transformed. These parts can play, create, connect. They're not protecting anymore because they don't need to—they feel safe. One client had a part she called "the artist" that could only emerge when she was deeply regulated. It literally required ventral vagal activation to exist.

In the sympathetic zone, we find the fighters and controllers. The inner critic that attacks to prevent external criticism. The perfectionist that stays in constant motion to avoid feeling. The angry protector that keeps people at distance. These parts maintain mobilization as their primary protection strategy. They believe safety comes from action, control, vigilance.

Down in dorsal vagal, we find the parts that protect through disconnection. The dissociator that takes us away when things get too intense. The nihilist that has given up hope. The sleepy part that just wants to check out. These parts use shutdown, numbing, and absence as protection. They've learned that when you can't fight or flee, disappearing is the only option.

Between zones, we might find parts that oscillate or guard the transitions. I had a client with a part that would panic whenever she started to feel good (moving from sympathetic to ventral) because good feelings had always preceded disappointment. Another had a part that would create crisis whenever she started to shut down (moving from ventral toward dorsal) because complete shutdown felt like death.

How Parts Interrupt Therapy: A Nervous System Perspective

We've all experienced it—a session is going well, the client is regulated and insightful, then suddenly something shifts. They become agitated, or spacey, or completely different. In IFS terms, a part has taken over. But through a Polyvagal lens, we can see this as an autonomic state shift triggered by a protective part that perceives danger.

According to research by Fisher on structural dissociation, different parts can trigger instant autonomic shifts. A client might be in ventral vagal, engaged in therapy, when something we say or do triggers a part that immediately shifts them to sympathetic activation or dorsal shutdown. The part doesn't just bring thoughts and feelings—it brings an entire autonomic state.

These interruptions often happen at precisely the moments when therapy is about to become effective. As we approach an exile (wounded part), protectors activate their defensive states. As we near a breakthrough, firefighters mobilize their emergency responses. What looks like resistance is actually parts shifting the nervous system to states where the threatening therapeutic work becomes impossible.

I learned to track these shifts somatically. With James, I could see his "angry protector" arriving—his jaw would tighten, his breathing would quicken, his hands would clench. This sympathetic activation would happen before he consciously knew the part was present. By naming the somatic shift first—"I notice your body just changed"— we could catch the part's activation early and work with it rather than being derailed by it.

Different parts use different autonomic strategies to interrupt therapy. Some flood the system with sympathetic activation— suddenly everything is urgent, crisis, chaos. Others trigger dorsal shutdown—suddenly the client can't think, can't feel, can't even remember why they're in therapy. Some parts oscillate between states so rapidly that the instability itself becomes the protection.

The 8 C's of Self and Polyvagal Correlates

Let's look deeper at how each of the 8 C's of Self corresponds to ventral vagal activation. According to research by Geller on therapeutic presence, these qualities emerge naturally when we're in a regulated state with access to our social engagement system.

Curiosity requires the openness and safety of ventral vagal. When we're curious, our nervous system is saying "this is interesting, not dangerous." In sympathetic, we're too focused on threat to be curious. In dorsal, we're too disconnected to care.

Compassion literally requires the care-giving system that's part of our social engagement complex. Research by Gilbert on compassion-focused therapy shows that compassion activates specific neural circuits associated with ventral vagal activation. You cannot access genuine compassion from a defensive state.

Clarity emerges when we're not clouded by the tunnel vision of sympathetic or the fog of dorsal. In ventral vagal, we can see the bigger picture, hold multiple perspectives, understand complexity. The prefrontal cortex stays online, allowing for the kind of reflection and integration that clarity requires.

Creativity needs the playfulness and flexibility of a regulated nervous system. According to research by Porges on play and social engagement, creativity emerges from the same neural platform as social connection. When we're in survival mode, we default to rigid, known patterns. Creativity requires the safety to explore the unknown.

Calm is perhaps the most obvious—it's the physiological state of ventral vagal itself. Not the flat calm of dorsal shutdown, but the alive, present calm of a regulated nervous system. It's calm with energy, peace with engagement.

Confidence comes from knowing we can handle what comes. This isn't the false confidence of a protective part but the grounded confidence of a nervous system that knows it can regulate, that has resources, that isn't alone.

Courage requires enough safety to take risks. According to research by Porges on the biological basis of courage, we need ventral vagal activation to face challenges without being overwhelmed. It's not the absence of fear but the presence of enough regulation to act despite fear.

Connectedness is the hallmark of ventral vagal—the social engagement system online, reaching for others, open to co-regulation. This isn't the desperate clinging of sympathetic or the false connection of fawning, but genuine, regulated connection.

The Integration That Heals

When we bring together IFS and Polyvagal Theory, we get a complete picture of healing. IFS shows us the multiplicity of the psyche—how we're made up of parts, each with its own story and protective role. Polyvagal Theory shows us the biological platform these parts operate from—the autonomic states that shape their perceptions and limit their options.

This integration helps us understand why some parts work is so difficult. We're not just dealing with psychological resistance—we're working with nervous system states that have been protecting someone for years or decades. A part that has maintained sympathetic vigilance since childhood doesn't just have a belief system about danger—it has an entire biological commitment to staying mobilized.

But this integration also gives us more precise ways to help. Instead of just talking to parts, we can help regulate the nervous system states they inhabit. Instead of just seeking Self, we can create the ventral vagal conditions for Self to emerge. Instead of fighting against protective parts, we can appreciate the autonomic states they've maintained for survival and help them discover that new states are now possible.

Most beautifully, this integration shows us that healing happens both psychologically and physiologically. As parts unburden and transform in IFS work, nervous system states shift and become more flexible. As we regulate autonomic states through Polyvagal-informed work, parts feel safer and become more willing to transform. The psychological and biological dance together, each supporting the other's movement toward wholeness.

Chapter 14: Clinical Applications of Polyvagal-Informed IFS

Rachel sat curled in my office chair, describing her inner world like a battlefield. "There's the one that screams at me to do better, the one that wants to burn everything down when I fail, and somewhere underneath, this tiny voice that just wants someone to care." Through an IFS lens, she was describing a harsh manager, a desperate firefighter, and an exiled child part. Through a Polyvagal lens, she was describing sympathetic hypervigilance protecting against sympathetic rage, both guarding against the dorsal collapse of a wounded child. The integration of these perspectives would transform her healing journey.

Working with parts through a Polyvagal lens isn't just about understanding them better—it's about working with them in ways that respect their biological reality. Each part inhabits a specific autonomic state for a reason. Each protective strategy emerged from nervous system wisdom. When we approach parts with this understanding, they feel seen not just psychologically but physiologically. They can begin to trust that we understand not just what they do but why their bodies needed them to do it.

This chapter explores how to actually work with different types of parts from a Polyvagal perspective. How do we approach a part that's stuck in sympathetic overdrive? What about one frozen in dorsal shutdown? How do we help parts and Self co-regulate internally? These aren't just theoretical questions—they're practical challenges that arise in every session when we're working with complex trauma.

Working with Hyperaroused Protector Parts

Hyperaroused protectors live in sympathetic activation. According to research by Van der Hart and colleagues on the theory of structural dissociation, these parts formed during moments of mobilization and continue to maintain that state. They're the inner critics, perfectionists, controllers—all the parts that try to protect through action, vigilance, and control.

The traditional IFS approach might involve asking these parts to step back so we can work with exiles. But from a Polyvagal perspective, asking a sympathetically activated part to step back is like asking someone in the middle of a fire to relax. The part's nervous system is screaming "DANGER!" and we're essentially saying "Could you ignore that for a moment?" No wonder they resist.

Instead, we need to first help regulate the sympathetic activation the part carries. I might say, "I can feel how activated this part is. Its body is really mobilized, isn't it? That must be exhausting, maintaining that level of vigilance all the time." This validates the somatic reality the part lives in. We're not just seeing its protective role—we're seeing the biological cost of maintaining that protection.

With Marcus's inner critic, we spent sessions just helping it discharge some of its sympathetic activation. We'd have the part imagine pushing against a wall, or running in place, or shaking out the tension. Not to get rid of the part, but to help its nervous system experience some relief from chronic mobilization. Only after several sessions of this did the part have enough regulation to even consider why it was so vigilant.

According to research by Ogden on sensorimotor approaches to trauma, working with the body first can make psychological work more effective. This is especially true for hyperaroused parts. They need to experience some physiological relief before they can access the reflection and perspective-taking necessary for transformation.

Sometimes these parts need to tell the story of when they first got activated. "When did you first have to be so vigilant? What was happening in the body then?" Often, they're still responding to a threat from decades ago, maintaining the same sympathetic activation that helped them survive that moment. Understanding this helps both therapist and client appreciate why the part can't just "calm down."

Approaching Hypoaroused and Dissociated Parts

Parts in dorsal shutdown present different challenges. According to research by Lanius on the neurobiology of dissociation, these states involve such profound deactivation that normal therapeutic engagement becomes impossible. These parts protect through absence—checking out, numbing, disappearing. How do you work with something that's barely there?

The key is gentle, gradual activation. Not sympathetic activation— we don't want to trigger fight or flight—but just enough mobilization to bring the part online. This might start with the tiniest movements. "Can this part feel anything in the body? Even numbness or heaviness?" We're looking for any sensation, any sign of life in the shutdown state.

With Jennifer's dissociative part, we started with temperature. Could the part notice warm or cold? Then texture—smooth or rough? Then movement—could it wiggle a finger? Each tiny activation was progress, slowly bringing the dorsal vagal state back toward the window of tolerance. It took months before this part had enough activation to even communicate why it protected through disappearing.

These parts often need to experience safety in the body before they can risk coming more fully online. According to research by Van der Kolk on body-based approaches to trauma, creating positive somatic experiences can help shift dorsal states. We might use weighted blankets for grounding, essential oils for sensory awakening, or very gentle movement to create mobilization without threat.

The therapist's regulated presence is crucial when working with shutdown parts. Our ventral vagal activation can help co-regulate the part toward more engagement. But we have to be careful not to be too energetic or enthusiastic, which can be overwhelming. Think of it like gently warming someone with hypothermia—too much heat too fast can be harmful.

The 5 P's and 6 F's Through a Polyvagal Lens

In IFS, we track certain patterns in how parts show up. The 5 P's describe how Self gets obscured: parts can be Protective, Proactive, Pervasive, Persistent, and Polarized. Through a Polyvagal lens, each of these patterns correlates with specific autonomic dynamics.

Protective parts maintain defensive autonomic states. They're not just protecting psychologically—they're maintaining sympathetic or dorsal states that once ensured survival. **Proactive** parts anticipate threat and shift the nervous system preemptively. They might trigger sympathetic activation at the slightest hint of danger. **Pervasive** parts flood the system with their autonomic state, making it hard to access any other state. **Persistent** parts maintain chronic activation or shutdown, unable to let the nervous system return to baseline. **Polarized** parts battle between opposite autonomic states—one pushing toward sympathetic, another toward dorsal, creating internal chaos.

The 6 F's describe protective strategies: Fight, Flight, Freeze, Fawn, Fold, and Faint. According to research by Kozlowska and colleagues on defense responses, each of these correlates with specific autonomic states. Fight and Flight are sympathetic mobilization. Freeze is the combination of sympathetic and dorsal activation—the body ready to act but immobilized. Fawn involves using the social engagement system defensively. Fold and Faint are progressive degrees of dorsal shutdown.

Understanding these patterns through a Polyvagal lens helps us work more effectively. A part using Fight isn't just angry—it's maintaining sympathetic mobilization for protection. A part using Freeze isn't just stuck—it's caught between competing autonomic states. This understanding helps us tailor interventions to the actual biological state rather than just the surface presentation.

Internal Co-Regulation Between Self and Parts

One of the most beautiful aspects of combining IFS and Polyvagal Theory is understanding how Self can co-regulate parts internally. Just as therapist and client co-regulate externally, Self and parts can co-regulate internally. According to research by Siegel on interpersonal neurobiology, the same principles that govern external relationships apply to internal relationships.

When a client accesses Self-energy (ventral vagal activation), that regulated state can begin to influence activated or shutdown parts. We might guide this explicitly: "Can your Self send some of that calm to the anxious part? Not to make it stop being anxious, just to let it know it's not alone." This is internal co-regulation—the ventral vagal state of Self offering regulation to parts in defensive states.

I teach clients to use their breath as a bridge for internal co-regulation. "Breathe toward the scared part. Let your breath carry Self-energy to it." This isn't just metaphorical—according to research by Porges on respiratory sinus arrhythmia, conscious breathing can shift autonomic states. The client is literally using breath to bring ventral vagal activation to sympathetic or dorsal parts.

113

Sometimes parts need to borrow Self's body awareness. A dissociated part might not be able to feel the body, but Self can. "Can Self share its awareness of your feet on the floor with the floating part?" This helps parts stuck in defensive states access the grounding and orientation that ventral vagal activation provides.

Internal co-regulation works both ways. Sometimes parts can help regulate each other. A part that knows how to be calm might help an anxious part. A part that can mobilize might help a shutdown part. We're facilitating not just dialogue between parts but autonomic regulation between different states.

Unburdening Through Nervous System Regulation

In IFS, unburdening is the process by which parts release the burdens they've carried—the pain, beliefs, and sensations from the past. Through a Polyvagal lens, we can see that parts also carry autonomic burdens—the frozen physiological states from trauma. True unburdening needs to address both psychological and physiological burdens.

According to research by Levine on somatic experiencing, trauma resolution requires completing interrupted defensive responses. Many parts are stuck mid-response—about to fight but couldn't, needing to run but trapped, starting to shut down but forced to stay present. The unburdening process can include letting these responses complete.

With Tom's protector part that carried rage from childhood abuse, unburdening involved first letting the part express the fight response that couldn't happen then. We had the part imagine pushing the abuser away, saying no, fighting back. The sympathetic activation could finally discharge. Only then could the part release the psychological burdens of shame and powerlessness.

For parts in dorsal shutdown, unburdening might involve grieving the collapse that had to happen. "This part had to shut down to survive. Can we honor that? Can it feel Self's compassion for how young you were, how overwhelming it was?" The combination of ventral vagal warmth from Self with acknowledgment of the dorsal state can help the part gradually release its frozen burden.

The elements used in IFS unburdening rituals—light, water, fire, earth, air—can be understood as supporting nervous system regulation. Light might represent ventral vagal clarity. Water might help discharge sympathetic activation. Earth might ground dorsal dissociation. We're not just using symbols—we're engaging somatic experiences that support autonomic shifts.

Precision and Compassion in Integration

When we bring Polyvagal awareness to IFS work, every intervention becomes more precise. We're not just working with parts as psychological entities—we're working with the nervous system states they inhabit and protect. This makes the work both more complex and more compassionate. Complex because we're tracking multiple levels simultaneously. Compassionate because we're seeing the biological wisdom in every protective strategy.

This integration also helps us understand why parts work can be so challenging. We're not just asking parts to change their minds— we're asking them to shift states they've maintained for survival. We're not just seeking psychological healing—we're facilitating biological reorganization at the deepest levels.

Most importantly, this approach honors both the multiplicity of the psyche and the unity of the nervous system. Yes, we have parts with different roles and perspectives. And yes, these parts share a nervous system that's always seeking safety and connection. By working with both levels, we can facilitate healing that's both psychologically meaningful and biologically regulating.

As you integrate these approaches, trust both the wisdom of parts and the intelligence of the nervous system. When a part resists, check what autonomic state it's protecting. When progress feels stuck, look for which nervous system patterns need attention. The combination of IFS's respect for internal multiplicity and Polyvagal Theory's understanding of biological states creates a framework for healing that honors the full complexity of human experience.

Chapter 15: Somatic Experiencing and Polyvagal Theory

The gazelle on the African savanna gets chased by a lion. It escapes, and within minutes, it's grazing peacefully again. No trauma, no PTSD, no years of therapy needed. How? Peter Levine watched nature documentaries for years, observing this phenomenon, and noticed something crucial: after the chase, the gazelle shakes. Its whole body trembles, discharging the massive sympathetic activation from the life-or-death encounter. Then it returns to baseline, ready to graze. Humans have the same capacity, but we've socialized ourselves out of it. We tell ourselves to "calm down," "get it together," "don't be dramatic." And in doing so, we trap the survival energy in our bodies, where it creates havoc for years or decades.

When Peter Levine's Somatic Experiencing meets Stephen Porges' Polyvagal Theory, we get a complete picture of trauma and healing. Levine shows us how trauma gets stuck in the body as incomplete defensive responses. Porges shows us the neurobiological platform these responses operate from. Together, they give us a map for helping the body complete what got interrupted and return to regulation.

These aren't competing theories—they're complementary lenses looking at the same phenomenon. Somatic Experiencing gives us the "what"—what needs to happen for trauma to resolve. Polyvagal Theory gives us the "why"—why the nervous system responds as it does and why certain interventions work. When we understand both, our clinical work becomes more precise, more effective, and more respectful of the body's inherent wisdom.

Peter Levine's Work and Stephen Porges' Theory: Complementary Approaches

According to research by Payne, Levine, and Crane-Godreau on somatic experiencing as trauma therapy, Levine's approach focuses on the body's innate capacity to heal from trauma through completing thwarted defensive responses. Meanwhile, Porges' work, as described in his foundational research on the polyvagal theory, explains the neurobiological substrates that make this healing possible.

Levine discovered that trauma isn't just about what happened to us—it's about what happened in our bodies during and after the event. When we face overwhelming threat, our nervous system mobilizes massive energy for survival. If we can fight or flee successfully, that energy gets discharged through action. But if we can't—if we're trapped, overpowered, or frozen—that energy gets stuck. The body remains in a state of activation or shutdown, even years after the danger has passed.

Porges' theory explains why this happens at a neurobiological level. When our neuroception detects life threat, our nervous system shifts into defensive states—sympathetic mobilization or dorsal vagal shutdown. These states are meant to be temporary, but trauma can lock them in place. The nervous system loses its flexibility, stuck in patterns that once ensured survival but now create suffering.

The beauty of combining these approaches is how they inform each other. Levine's clinical observations about how animals discharge trauma align perfectly with Porges' explanation of how the autonomic nervous system returns to baseline. Levine's emphasis on titration—working with small amounts of activation—makes sense through Porges' understanding of the window of tolerance. Levine's focus on completing interrupted defensive responses maps onto

118

Porges' description of how the nervous system moves through its evolutionary hierarchy.

I saw this powerfully with David, a car accident survivor. Through a Somatic Experiencing lens, his body was still braced for impact, muscles contracted, breath held. Through a Polyvagal lens, he was stuck in a mixed state—sympathetic activation (ready to act) combined with dorsal immobility (unable to act). The combination helped us understand both what his body needed (to complete the defensive response) and why it was stuck (caught between competing autonomic states).

Tracking Sensations and Autonomic Responses

Somatic Experiencing teaches us to track sensations as the language of the nervous system. According to research by Kuhfuß and colleagues on somatic experiencing for post-traumatic stress, this sensation-based approach can effectively address trauma without requiring detailed verbal processing. When we add Polyvagal awareness, we can read these sensations as communications about autonomic state.

Different sensations correlate with different autonomic states. Tingling, buzzing, or warmth often indicate sympathetic activation—the nervous system mobilizing energy. Heaviness, numbness, or coldness might signal dorsal shutdown. Flowing, spreading, or softening sensations often accompany the return to ventral vagal regulation. By tracking these sensations, we're essentially reading the nervous system's state moment by moment.

But here's what's crucial: we track sensations without trying to change them. This is what Levine calls "felt sense"—simply noticing what's present in the body without judgment or agenda. Through a Polyvagal lens, this makes perfect sense. The nervous system needs to be witnessed, not fixed. When we bring curious attention to sensation without trying to change it, we're offering the ventral vagal presence of the observing mind to whatever autonomic state is active.

Sarah would come to sessions completely disconnected from her body—classic dorsal shutdown. Traditional talk therapy went nowhere because she couldn't feel anything. So we started with the tiniest sensations. "Can you notice the temperature of your hands?" "What about the weight of your feet on the floor?" Each sensation we tracked was a small activation, gently bringing her nervous system back online. We weren't forcing change—we were inviting her body to tell its story through sensation.

The quality of sensation tells us about the state of the nervous system. Stuck, frozen sensations suggest incomplete responses waiting to complete. Moving, changing sensations indicate the nervous system actively processing. Rhythmic, flowing sensations often signal regulation returning. By tracking these qualities, we know whether to slow down, speed up, or simply witness what's unfolding.

Titration and Pendulation for Nervous System Regulation

Titration—working with small, manageable amounts of activation—is central to both Somatic Experiencing and Polyvagal-informed therapy. According to research by Brom and colleagues comparing body-focused therapy to other approaches, titrated somatic work can be more effective than cognitive approaches for certain trauma presentations. Through a Polyvagal lens, titration respects the window of tolerance, ensuring we don't overwhelm an already overwhelmed nervous system.

Think of titration like adding salt to soup. You add a little, taste, adjust. You don't dump the whole container in at once. Same with processing trauma—we touch the activation lightly, see how the nervous system responds, then decide whether to continue or pause.

This prevents retraumatization and builds the nervous system's capacity gradually.

Pendulation takes this further by consciously moving attention between activation and calm, between trauma and resource. Levine observed that the nervous system naturally pendulates—moving between states as part of its regulatory rhythm. Porges' theory explains this as the natural oscillation of the autonomic nervous system, constantly adjusting to internal and external conditions.

With Jennifer, who had medical trauma, even thinking about hospitals sent her into panic. So we pendulated. "Notice that tightness in your chest... now find somewhere in your body that feels okay, even a little okay... back to the chest—has it changed?... now back to the okay place." We were teaching her nervous system that activation doesn't have to be all-consuming, that there's always somewhere else to go.

Pendulation also happens between different autonomic states. Someone might pendulate between sympathetic activation and ventral vagal calm, gradually increasing their tolerance for activation while maintaining access to regulation. Or between dorsal shutdown and gentle mobilization, slowly coming back to life. The key is following the body's natural rhythm rather than forcing a particular outcome.

Releasing Thwarted Survival Energy Safely

According to research by Levine on the treatment of trauma, many symptoms arise from incomplete defensive responses—the body still holding the energy and patterns of actions that couldn't complete during the traumatic event. Polyvagal Theory helps us understand why: the nervous system remains in the defensive state associated with the incomplete response, unable to return to baseline.

Releasing this thwarted energy isn't about catharsis or dramatic emotional release. It's about giving the body permission to complete what got interrupted. This might be subtle—a slight pushing motion with the hands, a gentle turning of the head, a spontaneous deep breath. Or it might be more obvious—shaking, trembling, or heat moving through the body. Either way, we're allowing the nervous system to discharge the mobilization that got trapped.

Mark, a combat veteran, carried enormous rage that traditional anger management couldn't touch. Through somatic work, we discovered his body was still fighting—muscles tensed for combat, jaw clenched for battle. But the fight never got to complete. So we worked somatically. He pushed against the wall, imagining pushing away the danger. His body shook as years of thwarted fight response finally discharged. Afterward, for the first time in years, he felt calm.

But release needs to happen safely, within the window of tolerance. According to research by van der Kolk on body-based approaches to trauma, overwhelming discharge can retraumatize rather than heal. This is where Polyvagal awareness is crucial. We monitor the nervous system's capacity, ensuring enough ventral vagal regulation to integrate the discharge. If someone starts moving outside their window, we slow down, resource, regulate.

Sometimes the safest release is imaginal. The body doesn't always distinguish between real and imagined completion. A client who couldn't fight back during abuse might imagine pushing the abuser away, feeling the muscles engage without actual movement. The nervous system experiences completion without overwhelming activation.

The Felt Sense and Neuroception

Gendlin's concept of "felt sense"—the body's knowing beneath words and thoughts—intersects beautifully with Porges' concept of neuroception. According to research by Gendlin on focusing-oriented therapy, the felt sense is the body's implicit understanding of a situation, accessible through careful attention to subtle bodily sensations. Neuroception is the nervous system's unconscious detection of safety or danger. Together, they represent the body's wisdom operating below conscious awareness.

The felt sense often communicates what neuroception has detected. That vague uneasiness in your stomach might be neuroception picking up subtle threat cues. The warmth spreading through your chest might be neuroception recognizing safety. By attending to felt sense, we're essentially listening to what neuroception is telling us about our environment and state.

This has profound clinical implications. When a client says, "Something feels off, but I don't know what," they're describing felt sense detecting something neuroception has noticed. Instead of dismissing this as anxiety or paranoia, we can explore it somatically. "Where do you feel that 'off' feeling? What's its quality? Does it have a shape, a texture, a movement?" We're helping them decode their neuroception's message.

Amy had been in therapy for years, talking about her "trust issues" without much progress. When we started tracking felt sense, she noticed a particular sensation—a tightening in her throat—that appeared around certain people. As we explored this somatically, she realized this sensation had been her body's warning system since childhood, accurately detecting people who weren't safe. Her "trust issues" were actually her neuroception working perfectly, but she'd been taught to ignore it.

The Body's Wisdom in Integration

When we bring together Somatic Experiencing and Polyvagal Theory, we honor both the body's trauma and its wisdom. We understand that symptoms aren't pathology but incomplete responses waiting to complete. We see that healing isn't about getting rid of sensations but about allowing them to move, change, and resolve naturally.

This integration also helps us work more precisely. We can identify which autonomic state holds the incomplete response and what type of completion is needed. Sympathetic activation might need discharge through movement. Dorsal shutdown might need gentle mobilization. Mixed states might need careful differentiation. We're not just following sensation—we're understanding the neurobiological story it's telling.

Most importantly, this combination reminds us that the body knows how to heal. The gazelle doesn't need therapy because it allows its body to complete the natural cycle of activation and discharge. Humans have the same capacity; we've just forgotten how to access it. By combining Levine's attention to the body's natural healing responses with Porges' understanding of the nervous system's biological imperatives, we can help people remember what their bodies never forgot.

The work is gentle but profound. We're not forcing healing—we're creating conditions where the body's natural healing responses can emerge. We're not interpreting or analyzing—we're tracking and supporting what wants to happen. We're trusting the millions of years of evolution that gave us these remarkable nervous systems, designed not just to survive threat but to recover and thrive afterward.

Chapter 16: Body-Based Interventions for State Regulation

My client Rebecca sat in my office, hyperventilating, caught in a panic attack that wouldn't stop. Words weren't reaching her—she was too activated to process language. So I did something simple: I started breathing loudly, making my exhale longer than my inhale, exaggerating the sound. Within moments, her breathing began to match mine. Not because I told her to, but because nervous systems naturally sync up. Five minutes later, she was calm enough to talk. "How did you do that?" she asked. I hadn't done anything—her body remembered how to regulate itself once it had a pattern to follow.

Body-based interventions work because they speak directly to the nervous system in its own language—not words or thoughts but breath, movement, rhythm, and sensation. Through a Polyvagal lens, we understand that these interventions aren't just "coping skills" or "relaxation techniques." They're precise tools that shift autonomic states, build new neural pathways, and teach the nervous system that regulation is possible.

What makes body-based approaches so powerful is that they work even when the thinking brain is offline. When someone's in sympathetic overdrive or dorsal shutdown, the parts of the brain that process language and logic aren't fully available. But the body is always present, always breathing, always sensing. By working through the body, we can shift states even when talking about feelings is impossible.

Breathing Techniques for Vagal Tone Enhancement

According to research by Gerritsen and Band on breathing practices and the nervous system, conscious breathing directly influences autonomic state through multiple pathways. The vagus nerve, our primary parasympathetic pathway, is intimately connected with breathing. Every exhale activates the vagus, slowing heart rate. Every inhale temporarily suppresses it. By consciously manipulating our breathing, we're directly adjusting our autonomic state.

The simplest technique is extending the exhale. Research by Laborde and colleagues on heart rate variability shows that longer exhales relative to inhales increase vagal tone. Try it now—breathe in for four counts, out for six. Feel that subtle shift toward calm? That's your vagus nerve responding. For clients in sympathetic activation, this simple pattern can be a lifeline back to regulation.

But here's what's crucial: the breathing technique needs to match the person's current state. Someone in extreme sympathetic activation might not be able to slow their breathing immediately. Starting where they are—maybe quick breaths in and out—then gradually slowing, works better than forcing a calm pattern they can't access. It's like downshifting gears in a car; you can't go straight from fifth to first.

For clients in dorsal shutdown, different breathing is needed. They might need more activation first—slightly faster breathing to create mobilization. Breath of fire from yoga traditions, or simple quick inhales through the nose, can help shift from shutdown toward the window of tolerance. Once there's more activation, we can work toward regulated breathing.

I teach clients to find their own optimal breathing pattern. What feels regulating to one person might be activating to another. Sarah found that box breathing (in for 4, hold for 4, out for 4, hold for 4) helped her focus when dissociating. Marcus preferred rapid exhales to discharge sympathetic energy. There's no universal prescription—the body knows what it needs.

Movement Practices: Dance, Yoga, and Therapeutic Exercise

Movement is medicine for the nervous system, but not all movement affects autonomic states equally. According to research by Fonseca and colleagues on dance/movement therapy for trauma, rhythmic, expressive movement can help regulate autonomic states and process traumatic experience somatically. Through a Polyvagal lens, we can understand why different movements create different state shifts.

Vigorous movement—running, dancing, martial arts—helps discharge sympathetic activation. When the body is mobilized for fight or flight but can't act, that energy gets trapped. Vigorous movement completes the action, allowing the nervous system to discharge and return to baseline. It's not about exhaustion; it's about giving the mobilization somewhere to go.

Slow, mindful movement—tai chi, gentle yoga, walking meditation—helps shift from shutdown toward engagement without triggering sympathetic activation. According to research by Sullivan and colleagues on yoga and Polyvagal Theory, these practices can increase vagal tone while gently mobilizing the system. They're perfect for clients who need to come out of dorsal states without overwhelming their system.

Dance, particularly improvisational movement, allows the body to express what words can't. I worked with Maria, who couldn't talk about her trauma without dissociating. But when she danced it—showing through movement how it felt to be trapped, to fight, to collapse—her body told the story. The movement itself was healing, allowing her nervous system to complete responses that had been frozen for years.

127

The key is following the body's impulses rather than imposing structure. Sometimes the body needs to shake—literally trembling to discharge activation. Sometimes it needs to curl up—protecting and self-soothing. Sometimes it needs to push—completing a thwarted fight response. When we let the body move how it needs to, we're allowing the nervous system to regulate itself.

Creative Arts Therapies Through a Polyvagal Lens

According to research by Hass-Cohen and Carr on art therapy and neuroscience, creative expression activates neural networks that support regulation and integration. When we look at creative arts through a Polyvagal lens, we see that different art forms can shift autonomic states in specific ways.

Music has profound effects on the nervous system. According to research by Porges and Lewis on the listening project, certain frequencies and rhythms can directly influence vagal tone. Slow, melodic music with longer phrases tends to activate the ventral vagal system. Rhythmic drumming can help discharge sympathetic activation. Humming and singing create vibrations that literally stimulate the vagus nerve.

Visual art allows expression without words, crucial for experiences stored in implicit memory. The physical act of creating—the movement of drawing, the pressure of clay, the stroke of paint—provides bilateral stimulation and sensory input that can regulate the nervous system. Color choices often reflect autonomic states: reds and oranges might express sympathetic activation, blues and grays might indicate dorsal states, while greens and soft yellows often emerge with regulation.

I had a teenage client, Alex, who couldn't talk about their trauma but could draw it. The first drawings were all sharp angles and dark colors—pure sympathetic activation on paper. Over months, the drawings began to change. Curves appeared. Colors softened. By the end of treatment, they were drawing landscapes with both storms and sunshine—integration of all states, not just defense.

Drama therapy allows people to embody different states safely. Playing a powerful character might help someone access mobilization who's stuck in shutdown. Playing a calm character might give someone in chronic activation a taste of regulation. The "as if" quality of drama provides safety to explore states that feel too dangerous in real life.

Pranayama and Vagus Nerve Stimulation

Ancient yogic breathing practices, or pranayama, are essentially vagus nerve stimulation techniques that predated our understanding of the nervous system by thousands of years. According to research by Brown and Gerbarg on Sudarshan Kriya yoga, these practices can significantly impact autonomic regulation and stress resilience.

Alternate nostril breathing (Nadi Shodhana) balances the nervous system by alternating between sympathetic and parasympathetic activation. The left nostril connects more to parasympathetic activity, the right to sympathetic. By alternating, we're teaching the nervous system flexibility—the ability to shift states consciously rather than being stuck.

Bhramari (humming bee breath) creates vibrations that directly stimulate the vagus nerve. The humming sound resonates through the chest and throat, areas rich with vagal innervation. Clients often report immediate calming effects. It's particularly helpful for those who can't slow their breathing—they can hum at whatever speed feels comfortable while still getting vagal stimulation.

Modern vagus nerve stimulation techniques build on these ancient practices. Cold water on the face triggers the dive response, immediately activating the vagus nerve. Gargling vigorously stimulates vagal fibers in the throat. Even gentle pressure on the eyes (carefully done) can trigger vagal activation. These quick interventions can shift someone from panic to relative calm in moments.

But here's what's important: not every technique works for every nervous system. Someone with trauma involving suffocation might panic with breath retention practices. Someone with cold water trauma might find face immersion triggering. We always need to match the intervention to the person's history and current capacity.

Touch and Bodywork Considerations

Touch is complicated in trauma work. According to research by Field on touch therapy, appropriate touch can regulate the nervous system, reduce cortisol, and increase vagal tone. But for trauma survivors, touch can also be triggering, especially if their trauma involved boundary violations. Through a Polyvagal lens, we need to consider how different types of touch affect different autonomic states.

Self-touch is often the safest starting point. Teaching clients to place their own hands on their heart, to give themselves a butterfly hug (arms crossed, tapping alternately on upper arms), or to gently stroke their own arms gives them complete control over the touch. The nervous system can receive the regulating benefits without the potential threat of someone else's touch.

When professional bodywork is appropriate, the approach matters enormously. Gentle, predictable touch tends to activate ventral vagal states. Deep pressure (like deep tissue massage) might help discharge sympathetic activation but could trigger those prone to dissociation. Light, whisper-like touch might be soothing for some but triggering for others who need clearer boundaries.

I worked with a massage therapist who understood Polyvagal Theory. She would track her clients' autonomic states through their breathing, muscle tension, and skin temperature. If someone started shifting toward sympathetic (breathing quickening, muscles tensing), she'd lighten her touch and slow down. If someone was going dorsal (breathing becoming shallow, body becoming limp), she'd use slightly more pressure and movement to maintain engagement.

The key with any touch-based intervention is explicit consent and continuous checking. The nervous system needs to know it has choice and control. "Is this pressure okay?" "Would you like me to continue or pause?" These check-ins aren't just about consent—they're about keeping the social engagement system online, preventing the touch from triggering defensive responses.

The Body as the Gateway

Body-based interventions work because they bypass the stories, the defenses, the cognitive loops that keep us stuck. They speak directly to the part of us that knows how to heal—the body's inherent wisdom, developed over millions of years of evolution. When we breathe, move, create, and sense our way back to regulation, we're not learning something new. We're remembering something ancient.

Through a Polyvagal lens, we understand that these interventions aren't just about feeling better in the moment. They're about building new neural pathways, expanding the window of tolerance, and teaching the nervous system that it has options. Each time someone successfully uses breath to calm activation or movement to emerge from shutdown, they're proving to their nervous system that regulation is possible.

The beauty of body-based approaches is their accessibility. You don't need to understand trauma theory to breathe. You don't need insight to move. You don't need to remember your trauma to create art. The body can lead the way, and the nervous system will follow.

Most importantly, body-based interventions return agency to the person. After trauma, people often feel betrayed by their bodies— bodies that couldn't fight back, that froze, that still carry the trauma. But through these practices, they discover that their body isn't the enemy. It's been trying to protect them all along. And now, it can be their ally in healing.

Chapter 17: Integrative Somatic Approaches

The conference room was full of skeptical psychiatrists. I was presenting on integrating somatic approaches with traditional therapy, and the resistance was palpable. Then I asked them to try something simple: "Cross your arms. Now cross them the other way." The room filled with awkward laughter as these brilliant doctors struggled with this basic movement. "That discomfort you're feeling?" I said. "That's your nervous system encountering a pattern it doesn't recognize. Now imagine that happening with emotional regulation, with relationships, with feeling safe. That's trauma." The room got quiet. Bodies understand what minds sometimes resist.

Integrative somatic approaches recognize that healing trauma requires working with the whole person—body, mind, and nervous system together. It's not enough to just talk about trauma or just work with the body. We need approaches that weave together cognitive understanding, emotional processing, somatic awareness, and nervous system regulation. Through a Polyvagal lens, we can see how different modalities complement each other, each addressing different aspects of autonomic dysregulation.

What makes integration so powerful is that it meets people where they are. Some clients need to start with cognition because diving into the body feels too threatening. Others need to start somatically because words fail them. Some need creative expression because linear processing doesn't match their experience. When we have multiple approaches available and understand how each affects the nervous system, we can tailor treatment precisely to what each person needs.

Psychomotor Therapy and Polyvagal Integration

According to recent reviews, psychomotor therapy and other body- and movement-oriented approaches combine structured movement, cultivation of body awareness, and integration of emotional processing to support recovery from trauma (van de Kamp et al., 2019; van de Kamp et al., 2025).

.Through a Polyvagal lens, psychomotor therapy works because it engages multiple levels of the nervous system simultaneously—the cognitive brain through awareness, the emotional brain through expression, and the survival brain through movement.

Psychomotor therapy recognizes that trauma memories are encoded motorically—in movement patterns, postures, and muscular holding. That forward shoulder position might be a protection pattern from childhood. That inability to turn your back to the door might be a survival strategy from assault. These aren't just habits; they're nervous system programs running below consciousness.

Working psychomotorically means exploring these patterns experientially. Instead of talking about feeling trapped, we might explore what trapped feels like in the body. How would you move if you were trapped? What would you need to do to get free? As clients explore these movements, they often spontaneously complete interrupted defensive responses, allowing the nervous system to finally discharge what it's been holding.

I worked with James, whose body was locked in a perpetual brace position from a car accident. Traditional physical therapy helped somewhat, but the tension always returned. Through psychomotor work, we discovered his body was still bracing for an impact that happened five years ago. We worked with micro-movements—tiny rehearsals of getting out of the way, of protecting himself differently. Gradually, his nervous system learned the danger had passed, and the chronic tension began to release.

The integration with Polyvagal Theory helps us understand which movements support which states. Expansive movements—reaching up, opening arms wide—tend to activate ventral vagal states. Contractive movements—curling up, protecting the core—might trigger dorsal responses. By consciously working with movement qualities, we can help shift autonomic states while processing trauma material.

DBT Skills Through an Autonomic Lens

Dialectical Behavior Therapy's distress tolerance skills take on new meaning when viewed through a Polyvagal lens. According to research by Safer, and colleagues on integrating somatic approaches with DBT, understanding the autonomic basis of emotional dysregulation can enhance DBT's effectiveness. The skills aren't just cognitive strategies—they're nervous system interventions.

The TIPP skill (Temperature, Intense exercise, Paced breathing, Paired muscle relaxation) directly targets autonomic states. Cold temperature triggers the dive response, activating the vagus nerve. Intense exercise discharges sympathetic activation. Paced breathing regulates vagal tone. Muscle relaxation shifts from sympathetic tension to parasympathetic release. When clients understand they're not just "coping" but actually shifting their biology, the skills become more meaningful.

Distraction techniques work because they interrupt the neural loops maintaining dysregulation. When someone's in sympathetic overdrive, their attention narrows to threat. Distraction—counting backwards, naming objects, playing word games—requires enough cognitive resources that the nervous system has to shift states to comply. It's not avoiding; it's giving the nervous system a break from defense.

The "wise mind" concept in DBT correlates beautifully with ventral vagal activation. Emotion mind tends to be sympathetically driven—

reactive, intense, impulsive. Reasonable mind might actually be a dorsal strategy—disconnected from feeling, overly logical. Wise mind emerges when we have access to ventral vagal regulation—able to feel and think simultaneously.

Radical acceptance becomes easier to understand through a Polyvagal lens. It's not about giving up or not caring—it's about shifting from sympathetic fighting against reality to ventral vagal engagement with what is. The nervous system stops wasting energy on defensive responses to unchangeable situations, freeing resources for actual problem-solving.

Sensorimotor Psychotherapy Applications

According to research by Ogden and Fisher on sensorimotor psychotherapy, this approach specifically addresses how trauma disrupts sensorimotor processing—our ability to accurately sense our body and respond appropriately. Through a Polyvagal lens, we see that different autonomic states create different sensorimotor experiences.

In sympathetic activation, sensorimotor processing becomes biased toward threat detection. Every sensation might be interpreted as danger. The client who feels their racing heart and immediately thinks "heart attack" isn't being dramatic—their nervous system is interpreting sensation through a threat filter. Sensorimotor work helps differentiate between sensation and interpretation.

In dorsal states, sensorimotor processing might shut down entirely. Clients report feeling nothing, being numb, losing track of their body in space. This isn't psychological denial—it's the nervous system disconnecting from sensory input that was once overwhelming. Sensorimotor work gently reconnects awareness to sensation, building tolerance gradually.

The approach uses specific experiments to explore and reshape sensorimotor patterns. A client who collapses when discussing their trauma might experiment with staying upright, noticing what changes. Someone who can't make eye contact might practice brief glances, tracking what happens in their body. These aren't behavioral exercises—they're explorations of how different movements and postures affect autonomic state.

I worked with Linda, who would literally become smaller when discussing her childhood—shoulders hunching, spine curving, even her voice getting tiny. Through sensorimotor work, we explored what happened when she maintained her full height while talking about difficult memories. At first, it felt "wrong," even dangerous. But gradually, her nervous system learned that she could be full-sized and still safe. The trauma memories didn't change, but her body's response to them did.

Clinical Somatic Education and Pandiculation

Pandiculation is what animals do naturally when they wake up—that stretching, yawning, contracting, and releasing. It's not stretching in the traditional sense; it's a specific sequence that resets the gamma motor system, which controls baseline muscle tone. When trauma creates chronic tension patterns, pandiculation can help release them at a neurological level.

The process involves three phases: conscious contraction of already-tight muscles (meeting the tension), slow conscious release (showing the nervous system how to let go), and complete relaxation (allowing a new baseline). This sequence speaks directly to the nervous system, saying "this defensive contraction is voluntary, and I can release it voluntarily."

Through a Polyvagal lens, pandiculation makes perfect sense. Chronic muscle tension often represents incomplete defensive responses—the body still ready to fight or flee. By consciously

137

contracting and then releasing, we're completing the response, allowing the nervous system to return to baseline. It's like finally finishing a sentence that's been half-spoken for years.

I teach clients simple pandiculation exercises they can do anywhere. When they notice tension building, they can consciously contract those muscles slightly more, then slowly release. It's empowering—instead of being victims of their tension, they become active participants in their regulation.

Trauma-Sensitive Yoga Practices

According to research by van der Kolk and colleagues on trauma-sensitive yoga, this modified approach to yoga specifically addresses the needs of trauma survivors. Through a Polyvagal lens, traditional yoga might actually be triggering—certain poses might activate defensive responses, the emphasis on proper form might trigger perfectionism, and the teacher's adjustments might violate boundaries.

Trauma-sensitive yoga makes several crucial modifications. Language is invitational rather than commanding—"when you're ready, you might explore" rather than "now do this." Choice is emphasized constantly—multiple options for every pose, permission to skip anything, encouragement to listen to their body over the instructor. Touch is generally avoided unless explicitly requested.

Different yoga practices affect autonomic states differently. Vigorous vinyasa might help discharge sympathetic activation but could overwhelm someone already activated. Gentle restorative yoga might support ventral vagal activation but could trigger someone prone to dissociation. Yin yoga's long holds might allow processing but could trap someone in uncomfortable sensation.

The genius of trauma-sensitive yoga is that it rebuilds interoception—awareness of internal sensation—which trauma often

138

disrupts. According to research by Mehling and colleagues on body awareness, improved interoception correlates with better emotional regulation. By gently guiding attention to sensation without judgment, yoga helps rebuild the connection between body and awareness.

Most importantly, trauma-sensitive yoga returns agency to the practitioner. After trauma, people often feel their body betrayed them or was taken from them. Yoga practiced this way says, "This is your body. You choose how to move it. You decide what feels right." Every choice to modify or skip a pose is a small reclamation of autonomic autonomy.

The Power of Integration

When we integrate somatic approaches with Polyvagal awareness, something profound happens. We stop seeing techniques as separate tools and start understanding them as different ways of speaking to the nervous system. DBT skills become somatic interventions. Yoga becomes nervous system regulation. Movement becomes trauma processing. Everything works together because it's all affecting the same biological system.

This integration also helps us understand why different approaches work for different people at different times. Someone in chronic sympathetic activation might need discharge-focused work initially—intense movement, emotional expression, maybe even EMDR. Someone in chronic dorsal shutdown might need gentle activation first—basic sensorimotor awareness, supported yoga, careful titration of sensation.

The key is flexibility and responsiveness. We're not applying protocols; we're responding to the nervous system in front of us. Today's intervention might not work tomorrow. What helps one person might trigger another. By understanding the autonomic effects of different approaches, we can adjust moment by moment, always working at the edge of the window of tolerance.

Most beautifully, integrative somatic approaches honor the wholeness of human experience. Trauma affects everything—body, mind, spirit, relationships. Healing needs to address all these levels. When we combine cognitive understanding, emotional processing, somatic awareness, and nervous system regulation, we're not just treating symptoms. We're facilitating a return to wholeness, to the full range of human experience that trauma truncated.

As you explore these integrative approaches, trust your observations. Watch how different interventions affect autonomic states. Notice what combinations work well together. The nervous system will tell you what it needs if you know how to listen. And remember—integration isn't about doing everything at once. It's about having multiple ways to support healing and knowing when to use each one.

Chapter 18: Complex Trauma and Developmental Applications

The seven-year-old boy sat in my office, completely still. Not the stillness of calm, but the frozen watchfulness of a child whose nervous system had learned that being noticed meant danger. His foster mother had brought him in for "behavioral problems," but what I saw wasn't a problem child—it was a nervous system shaped by years of unpredictability, neglect, and fear. When I moved too quickly reaching for a toy, he flinched. When I spoke too loudly, he shut down. His body was telling the story of developmental trauma more clearly than any words could.

Complex trauma doesn't just affect individuals—it ripples through families, communities, and generations. It shapes how veterans come home from war, how children grow up in chaotic households, how entire cultures respond to historical wounds. Through a Polyvagal lens, we can see that complex trauma isn't just about multiple bad experiences. It's about how repeated exposure to threat and the absence of co-regulation fundamentally alter the developing nervous system's architecture.

Working with complex trauma requires understanding that we're not just treating symptoms or even traumatic memories. We're working with nervous systems that developed differently, that learned to prioritize survival over growth, protection over connection. These adaptations were brilliant for surviving unsurvivable situations, but they create profound challenges when the danger has passed and the person is trying to build a life worth living.

Working with Developmental Trauma and Attachment Wounds

According to research by Schore on affect regulation and the origin of the self, early relational trauma fundamentally alters how the nervous system develops. The infant brain requires consistent co-regulation from caregivers to develop its own regulatory capacity. When that co-regulation is absent, inconsistent, or actively harmful, the nervous system develops along different lines—hypervigilant, quick to shut down, or oscillating wildly between states.

Developmental trauma creates what we might call a "narrow window from the start." These nervous systems never had the safety to develop a wide tolerance for stress. They're like buildings constructed on shaky foundations—functional, but requiring constant energy to stay stable. Through a Polyvagal lens, we see that these children didn't develop robust ventral vagal capacity because they rarely experienced the safety that builds it.

The attachment system and autonomic nervous system are intimately linked. Secure attachment develops when a child experiences consistent co-regulation—their distress is met with soothing, their joy with engagement, their needs with responsiveness. This repeated experience builds neural pathways for self-regulation. But in insecure attachment, different patterns emerge. Anxious attachment might correlate with chronic sympathetic activation—always seeking, never quite safe. Avoidant attachment might involve premature autonomic self-sufficiency—shutting down needs to avoid disappointment. Disorganized attachment often involves rapid oscillation between states—the caregiver is both source of comfort and threat.

Working with these wounds requires patience that goes beyond what traditional therapy demands. Sarah, a thirty-five-year-old survivor of childhood neglect, would dissociate the moment she felt any

142

emotional warmth from me. Her nervous system had learned that connection led to abandonment, so dorsal shutdown was protection against the pain of lost connection. We spent months just building tolerance for brief moments of co-regulation—five seconds of eye contact, a slight smile, a gentle "I'm glad you're here." Each micro-moment was building new neural pathways, teaching her nervous system that connection could be safe.

According to research by Perry and Szalavitz on developmental trauma, the brain develops sequentially, and healing needs to follow the same sequence. We can't just jump to cognitive processing with someone whose brainstem and limbic system are still alarmed. We need to work bottom-up, establishing safety in the body first, then emotional regulation, then cognitive integration. It's like building a house—you need a foundation before walls, walls before a roof.

Veterans and Combat-Related PTSD

Combat trauma presents unique challenges for the nervous system. According to research by Bremner on traumatic stress from a neurocircuitry perspective, combat involves repeated exposure to life threat while requiring continued functioning. The nervous system can't simply shut down or flee—it has to stay functional while experiencing extreme threat. This creates complex adaptations that don't simply resolve when the soldier comes home.

Veterans often describe feeling like they left part of themselves in the war zone. Through a Polyvagal lens, this makes perfect sense. Part of their nervous system is still there, still in combat mode, still scanning for IEDs and sniper fire. Their neuroception was trained to detect threats that civilian life doesn't present, but the detection system doesn't have an off switch.

The warrior culture adds another layer. Soldiers are trained to push through, to not show weakness, to protect others at all costs. These are sympathetic-dominant strategies that become identity, not just

143

behavior. Asking a veteran to "relax" or "let go" isn't just challenging their nervous system—it's challenging everything they were trained to be.

I worked with Marcus, a Marine with three deployments to Afghanistan. Traditional PTSD treatment had failed because every time he started to relax in therapy, his nervous system would scream "danger!" In combat, letting your guard down could get you and your buddies killed. His hypervigilance wasn't pathology—it was trained survival. We had to work differently, respecting his nervous system's wisdom while slowly teaching it to recognize the difference between combat zones and home.

We started with movement—boxing, running, activities that honored his need for mobilization while providing discharge. Then we worked on what I call "tactical relaxation"—maintaining alertness while reducing tension. Only after months of this could we begin to introduce true ventral vagal states. His nervous system needed to learn gradually that standing down didn't mean death.

Children and Adolescents: Age-Appropriate Interventions

Working with young nervous systems requires understanding that they're not just small adult nervous systems—they're developing systems with different capacities and needs. According to research by Blaustein and Kinniburgh on treating traumatic stress in children and adolescents, interventions need to match developmental capacity while building missing skills.

Young children can't tell you they're dysregulated—they show you. Tantrums might be sympathetic overwhelm. Withdrawal might be dorsal shutdown. "Defiance" might be a nervous system that can't tolerate the vulnerability of compliance. We need to read behavior as nervous system communication and respond accordingly.

Play becomes a crucial intervention because it's the natural language of childhood. A child might not be able to talk about their trauma, but they can play it out with dolls, draw it in pictures, or dance it in movement. Through play, we can see which autonomic states dominate and help build regulation without requiring cognitive processing they're not capable of.

I worked with eight-year-old Jamie, who'd witnessed domestic violence. He couldn't sit still, constantly moved, and had been labeled ADHD. But through a Polyvagal lens, I saw a nervous system stuck in sympathetic activation, ready to run at any moment. Instead of trying to calm him, we played "racing games" where he could run, then "sleeping games" where we practiced being very still. We were teaching his nervous system to move between states consciously, building flexibility.

Adolescents present unique challenges because their nervous systems are undergoing massive reorganization. The teenage brain is pruning neural connections and strengthening others, all while dealing with hormonal storms and social pressures. Trauma during this period can derail development in profound ways. According to research by Teicher and Samson on childhood maltreatment and brain development, trauma during adolescence can alter the trajectory of neural development, affecting regulation capacity into adulthood.

Neurodivergent Populations and Adapted Approaches

Neurodivergent individuals—those with autism, ADHD, sensory processing differences, and other neurological variations—often have unique autonomic patterns that require adapted approaches. According to research by Porges and colleagues on autism and the autonomic nervous system, many autistic individuals have differences in vagal tone and autonomic flexibility that affect their response to standard interventions.

Sensory sensitivities in autism often reflect autonomic dysregulation. What seems like a minor sensory input to a neurotypical nervous system might trigger massive defensive responses in an autistic nervous system. The fluorescent lights that others barely notice might trigger sympathetic activation. The texture of certain foods might trigger dorsal shutdown. We need to respect these as real nervous system responses, not behavioral problems.

ADHD involves differences in autonomic regulation that go beyond attention. According to research by Bellato and colleagues on autonomic function in ADHD, many individuals with ADHD have lower baseline arousal and need more stimulation to feel regulated. What looks like hyperactivity might be attempts to achieve an optimal arousal state. Movement isn't the problem—it's the solution their nervous system has found.

Working with neurodivergent clients requires flexibility in our approaches. Traditional sitting-still therapy might be dysregulating for someone whose nervous system needs movement to focus. Eye contact expectations might trigger defensive responses in autistic clients. We need to adapt our environments and interventions to match their nervous system needs, not force them to adapt to neurotypical expectations.

Alex, an autistic teenager, would shut down completely in traditional therapy. But when we met while walking, with parallel rather than face-to-face interaction, they could engage. The movement regulated their nervous system, the side-by-side positioning reduced social threat, and the predictable route provided safety. Their insights were brilliant once their nervous system felt safe enough to share them.

Cultural Trauma and Collective Nervous System Healing

Trauma doesn't just affect individuals—it affects entire communities and cultures. According to research by Menakem on racialized trauma, historical and ongoing oppression creates collective nervous system patterns that pass through generations. The hypervigilance of communities under threat, the shutdown of those whose voices have been silenced, the dysregulation of disconnection from cultural roots—these are collective autonomic adaptations to collective trauma.

Cultural trauma requires us to think beyond individual nervous systems to collective co-regulation. How do communities heal together? How do cultural practices support nervous system regulation? According to research by Wendt and colleagues on cultural concepts of trauma and healing, many indigenous and non-Western cultures have long understood what Polyvagal Theory now explains—that healing happens in relationship, through rhythm, through collective practices that regulate nervous systems together.

Drumming circles, group singing, collective dancing—these aren't just cultural expressions but nervous system interventions. The shared rhythm synchronizes nervous systems. The collective voice activates social engagement systems. The movement together discharges activation while building connection. These practices intuitively use Polyvagal principles that Western therapy is just beginning to understand.

Working with cultural trauma requires humility and recognition that Western therapy models might not be appropriate or sufficient. Maria, a refugee from Central America, found individual therapy helpful but incomplete. It wasn't until she joined a support group with other Spanish-speaking refugees, where they could share stories in their language, with their cultural expressions of grief and resilience, that her nervous system could truly begin to heal. The collective co-regulation of shared experience provided something individual therapy couldn't.

Adapting to Complexity

Working with complex trauma and diverse populations requires us to expand our understanding of what healing looks like. The goal isn't always individual symptom reduction—it might be family reconnection, community healing, or cultural reclamation. The nervous system doesn't exist in isolation; it's shaped by and shapes the systems around it.

This work also requires us to examine our own assumptions about what regulation looks like. A calm, quiet nervous system might be the goal for some, but for others, vibrant expressiveness might be regulation. What looks like dysregulation through one cultural lens might be healthy expression through another. We need to be careful not to pathologize differences or impose our own nervous system patterns as the standard.

Most importantly, working with complex trauma requires hope grounded in biology. Yes, early trauma shapes nervous system development. Yes, repeated trauma creates deep patterns. But neuroplasticity continues throughout life. New experiences can build new neural pathways. Safe relationships can repair attachment wounds. The nervous system's fundamental drive toward connection and regulation never disappears—it just needs the right conditions to emerge.

As we work with these complex applications, we're not just treating individuals—we're contributing to the healing of families, communities, and cultures. Each nervous system that finds regulation becomes a resource for others. Each person who learns to co-regulate can offer that gift to those around them. The ripples extend far beyond the therapy room.

Chapter 19: Group and Systems Applications

The therapy group sat in uncomfortable silence. Eight trauma survivors, each locked in their own nervous system state—some visibly agitated, others checked out, a few frozen in hypervigilance. Then something shifted. One member took a deep breath, audibly sighing. Without planning, another member matched it. Then another. Within minutes, the entire group was breathing together, not because I instructed it but because nervous systems naturally seek co-regulation when it's available. That moment changed everything about how I understood group work.

Groups aren't just collections of individuals—they're living systems with their own autonomic dynamics. When we understand groups through a Polyvagal lens, we see that collective nervous system states emerge, spread, and shift in predictable ways. A single activated member can trigger a cascade of sympathetic arousal through the group. But equally, a regulated presence can offer an anchor that helps everyone settle. This isn't just emotional contagion—it's biological synchronization at the deepest level.

The same principles apply to families, organizations, even entire communities. Wherever nervous systems gather, they influence each other. Trauma ripples through systems, creating patterns of dysregulation that can persist for generations. But healing can ripple too. When we understand how to work with collective nervous system dynamics, we can facilitate healing that extends far beyond individual therapy rooms.

Group Therapy Through a Polyvagal Lens

According to research by Flores and Porges on group therapy and attachment, groups provide unique opportunities for nervous system healing that individual therapy cannot replicate. In a group, members experience multiple nervous systems simultaneously, creating a rich field of co-regulatory possibilities. But this same richness can be overwhelming without careful attention to autonomic states.

Group composition matters enormously from a Polyvagal perspective. Too many members in sympathetic activation creates a chaotic field that prevents regulation. Too many in dorsal shutdown creates a heavy, disconnected atmosphere. The ideal group has enough regulated presence to hold the activation and enough activation to mobilize the shutdown. It's a delicate balance that requires constant attunement.

The physical setup of group space directly impacts collective nervous system states. Circle formations allow everyone to see everyone—maximizing social engagement but potentially triggering for those who need less visibility. Rows might feel safer but reduce co-regulatory possibilities. I often let groups experiment with different configurations, noticing how arrangement affects their collective state.

Opening rituals become crucial for establishing collective regulation. We might start with a minute of silent breathing together, feeling into the shared space. Or a simple check-in using body sensations: "tight shoulders," "heavy chest," "buzzy stomach." This isn't just sharing—it's nervous systems beginning to synchronize, finding a collective rhythm.

The power of group work through a Polyvagal lens is that members can borrow regulation from each other. When Tom panics, he can feel Sarah's calm presence beside him. When Lisa dissociates, she can anchor to the group's collective engagement. The group becomes a larger nervous system that can hold more than any individual system could.

Family Systems and Co-Regulation Dynamics

Families are co-regulation systems, whether functional or dysfunctional. According to research by Lunkenheimer and colleagues on parent-child coregulation, family members' autonomic states constantly influence each other, creating patterns that can support or undermine regulation. Through a Polyvagal lens, family dysfunction often reflects collective nervous system dysregulation rather than individual pathology.

In healthy families, there's what I call "regulatory flexibility"— different members can take turns being the regulated presence when others are activated. Dad might be the calm anchor when mom is stressed, mom might provide soothing when the kids are overwhelmed, even children can offer playful regulation when adults are too serious. This flexibility creates resilience.

But in traumatized families, patterns become rigid. Maybe dad's PTSD keeps him in chronic sympathetic activation, triggering mom's anxiety, which activates the older child's perfectionism, which triggers the younger child's withdrawal. Everyone's responding to everyone else's dysregulation, creating escalating cycles that no one knows how to interrupt.

I worked with the Martinez family—two parents, three kids, all traumatized by a house fire. In family sessions, you could watch dysregulation spread like wildfire. Dad would tense up, mom would start talking rapidly, the teenager would get angry, the middle child would space out, the youngest would start acting out. Within minutes, the room was chaos. Individual therapy hadn't helped because they went home to the same dysregulated system.

We started with simple co-regulation exercises. Having them breathe together. Pass a rhythm around the circle. Make eye contact with appreciation. These weren't just activities—they were teaching the family system new patterns. Gradually, they learned to recognize when the family nervous system was escalating and how to interrupt it. They developed signals—dad would say "yellow light" when he felt activation building, mom would suggest "breathing break," the kids learned to ask for "family hugs" when overwhelmed.

Organizational and Workplace Applications

Workplaces are nervous system environments that profoundly impact employee wellbeing and performance. According to research by Heaphy and Dutton on positive social interactions at work, the quality of interpersonal connections directly affects physiological stress responses. Through a Polyvagal lens, toxic workplaces are environments of chronic autonomic dysregulation, while healthy workplaces support nervous system regulation.

Leadership sets the autonomic tone. A chronically activated leader—always urgent, always crisis-mode—creates a sympathetically-charged environment where everyone stays on edge. A disconnected leader might create an environment of dorsal withdrawal where innovation and engagement shut down. But a regulated leader who maintains ventral vagal presence even during challenges creates safety that allows others to stay regulated too.

Meeting dynamics reveal collective nervous system patterns. That meeting where everyone talks over each other? That's sympathetic chaos with no co-regulation. The meeting where everyone checks out? That's collective dorsal withdrawal. But meetings can become co-regulatory experiences with simple modifications. Starting with a moment of settling. Having a talking stick that slows down reactive responses. Building in movement breaks when activation builds.

I consulted with a tech startup where burnout was rampant. Through a Polyvagal lens, the entire organization was stuck in sympathetic overdrive—everything urgent, no rest, constant mobilization. We implemented what I called "regulation rhythms"—predictable patterns of activation and rest. Focused work sprints followed by genuine breaks. High-intensity meetings followed by walking meetings. Deadline pushes followed by celebration and recovery. The productivity actually increased when the nervous systems had time to regulate.

Physical workspace impacts collective autonomic states. Open offices might promote collaboration but can trigger constant vigilance. Private offices might feel safer but can increase disconnection. According to research by Sander and colleagues on office design and stress, environments that offer both connection and retreat possibilities best support nervous system regulation. We need spaces for co-regulation and spaces for self-regulation.

Community Healing and Collective Resilience

Communities, like individuals, can experience collective trauma that dysregulates entire populations. According to research by Pinderhughes and colleagues on community trauma and resilience, traumatic events—whether acute like natural disasters or chronic like systemic oppression—create community-wide autonomic adaptations.

After collective trauma, communities often show predictable patterns. Some become hypervigilant, with everyone in sympathetic activation, suspicious and reactive. Others collapse into collective dorsal withdrawal—hopeless, disconnected, unable to mobilize. Many oscillate between extremes, swinging from passionate mobilization to exhausted withdrawal.

153

But communities also have unique resources for collective healing. Rituals, traditions, and cultural practices often contain embedded co-regulation strategies. According to research by Hobfoll and colleagues on community resilience, communities that maintain cultural practices and social connections show better recovery from collective trauma.

I witnessed this after a school shooting in a small town. The immediate response was sympathetic chaos—anger, fear, desperate action. Then came dorsal collapse—numbness, withdrawal, isolation. But slowly, the community's natural co-regulation resources emerged. Prayer circles for those who found comfort in faith. Community dinners where people could be together without having to talk. A memorial garden where people could move between solitude and connection.

The key was respecting different nervous system needs while maintaining collective connection. Some needed to talk; others needed silence. Some needed action; others needed stillness. But by creating multiple ways to be together, the community could hold its diversity of responses while still co-regulating.

Training and Supervision Considerations

Training therapists to work with Polyvagal Theory requires more than intellectual understanding—it requires embodied learning. According to research by Geller and Porges on therapeutic presence, therapists' own nervous system regulation directly impacts their clinical effectiveness. We can't teach what we don't embody.

Supervision through a Polyvagal lens focuses not just on interventions but on the supervisor-supervisee nervous system dynamics. Is the supervisee activated when discussing certain clients? Do they dissociate when exploring their own triggers? The supervision relationship becomes a laboratory for developing co-regulatory skills that supervisees can then offer their clients.

Training programs need to include somatic components. It's not enough to read about autonomic states—trainees need to feel them, recognize them, learn to shift between them. This might feel uncomfortable for therapists trained in cognitive approaches, but embodied learning is essential for Polyvagal-informed practice.

I run training groups where we practice co-regulation before learning theory. Participants experience what it's like to help regulate another's nervous system and to have their own system regulated by others. They learn to recognize their own triggers and resources. Only after this embodied experience do we add theoretical understanding.

Burnout prevention becomes central when training therapists to work with trauma. According to research by Porges and Buczynski on therapist self-care, maintaining our own nervous system regulation isn't just personal wellness—it's professional responsibility. We need to teach therapists to recognize their own autonomic patterns and develop robust self-regulation practices.

Systems Thinking for Nervous System Healing

When we expand our view from individual to collective nervous systems, we see that healing is always relational, always embedded in larger systems. The traumatized child exists within a family system, which exists within a school system, which exists within a community system. Dysregulation at any level affects all levels. But equally, regulation at any level can ripple outward.

This systems perspective changes how we intervene. Instead of just treating the identified patient, we might work with the family's co-regulation patterns. Instead of just offering individual therapy, we might create group experiences that build collective regulation. Instead of just focusing on symptom reduction, we might address the environmental factors that perpetuate dysregulation.

155

Working with systems requires humility. We can't control how nervous systems influence each other, but we can create conditions that support co-regulation. We can't force collective healing, but we can facilitate experiences that make it possible. We can't eliminate all sources of dysregulation, but we can build resilience through connection.

The beauty of systems work is that small changes can have large effects. One regulated presence in a chaotic family can begin to shift the entire system. One safe relationship in a traumatized community can begin to restore trust. One organization that prioritizes nervous system health can model what's possible for others.

As we apply Polyvagal Theory to groups and systems, we're participating in something larger than individual healing. We're contributing to the evolution of human systems toward greater regulation, connection, and resilience. Each group that learns to co-regulate, each family that breaks cycles of trauma, each community that heals together—they all contribute to a more regulated world. And in a world facing collective challenges that require collective responses, this work has never been more important.

Chapter 20: Building Your Polyvagal-Informed Practice

The email arrived on a Tuesday afternoon. "I've been reading about Polyvagal Theory," my colleague wrote, "and I want to incorporate it into my practice. But I just realized I've been accidentally triggering my clients' nervous systems for years. Their faces when I sat behind the desk, the way they flinched when I took notes, their shutdown when I pushed for emotional expression—it all makes sense now. How do I rebuild my practice with this awareness without feeling like everything I've done before was wrong?"

Building a Polyvagal-informed practice isn't about throwing away everything you know—it's about adding a biological lens that makes your existing skills more precise and effective. Every theoretical orientation, every intervention you've learned can be enhanced by understanding the autonomic platform it operates from. But this integration requires thoughtfulness about ethics, documentation, outcomes, and our own nervous system health as practitioners.

The shift to working with nervous system states rather than just symptoms or cognitions fundamentally changes how we conceptualize treatment. We're not just reducing anxiety or processing trauma—we're helping nervous systems learn new patterns of regulation. This biological focus doesn't replace psychological understanding; it deepens it. When we understand the autonomic underpinnings of mental health challenges, our interventions become more targeted, our presence more attuned, and our outcomes more sustainable.

Ethical Considerations and Scope of Practice

Working with the nervous system raises important ethical questions. According to research by Wylie and Turner on integrating neuroscience into psychotherapy practice, therapists need to carefully consider their competence when incorporating somatic and neurobiological interventions. Just reading about Polyvagal Theory doesn't make us somatic therapists, and understanding nervous system states doesn't mean we should attempt interventions beyond our training.

The scope of practice issue is crucial. A talk therapist who understands Polyvagal Theory can use that knowledge to create safety, track states, and adjust their approach. But implementing specific somatic interventions requires appropriate training. Teaching breathing exercises might be within scope, but working with complex trauma through body-based methods might require additional certification. According to research by Ogden and Fisher on sensorimotor psychotherapy training, competent somatic work requires supervised practice, not just theoretical knowledge.

Informed consent takes on new dimensions when working with nervous system states. Clients need to understand that we'll be paying attention to their body's responses, not just their words. They need to know that healing might involve feeling sensations or emotions that have been shut down. Some clients find body awareness triggering, and we need to respect that. I always explain, "I'll be noticing things like changes in your breathing or posture because these tell us about your nervous system state. Is that okay with you?"

The power differential in therapy is magnified when working with autonomic states because we're often tracking things clients aren't consciously aware of. Saying "I notice your breathing just changed"

158

can feel invasive if not handled sensitively. We need to be transparent about what we're observing and why, always maintaining the client's autonomy and choice about how to proceed.

There's also an ethical imperative to work within the client's window of tolerance. According to research by Siegel on the developing mind, pushing someone beyond their regulatory capacity can retraumatize rather than heal. Just because we can trigger a state shift doesn't mean we should. The nervous system's protective responses deserve respect, even when they're causing suffering.

Documentation and Treatment Planning

Documentation from a Polyvagal perspective requires new language and frameworks. Instead of just noting "client appeared anxious," we might document "client presented in sympathetic activation: rapid speech, shallow breathing, scanning the room, difficulty maintaining eye contact." This specificity helps track progress and informs treatment planning.

Treatment plans need to include autonomic goals alongside psychological ones. Rather than just "reduce anxiety symptoms," we might target "increase capacity to recognize and down-regulate from sympathetic activation within 10 minutes" or "develop three reliable methods for shifting from dorsal withdrawal to ventral vagal engagement." These concrete, measurable goals help track nervous system changes over time.

I've developed a documentation template that includes autonomic state mapping. For each session, I note: starting state (sympathetic, dorsal, ventral, or mixed), state shifts during session, triggers observed, resources that helped regulation, and ending state. Over time, patterns emerge that inform treatment. Maybe the client always arrives activated but settles after 15 minutes. Maybe they shut down when discussing family but mobilize when talking about work.

Progress notes benefit from Polyvagal awareness. Instead of "processed trauma," we might write "client able to discuss traumatic event while maintaining window of tolerance, using breathing to regulate when approaching sympathetic activation." This documents not just what was discussed but the nervous system's capacity to hold the material.

According to research by Cook and colleagues on complex trauma treatment, documentation should track not just symptom reduction but increased flexibility and resilience. Are state shifts happening more smoothly? Is the window of tolerance expanding? Can the client recognize states and implement regulation strategies independently? These process measures often show progress before symptoms significantly decrease.

Measuring Outcomes and Tracking Progress

Traditional outcome measures might miss nervous system changes. Someone's anxiety scores might remain high even as their capacity to regulate that anxiety improves dramatically. According to research by Kearney and colleagues on treatment outcome assessment, multi-modal evaluation that includes physiological measures provides a more complete picture.

Heart rate variability (HRV) offers an objective measure of autonomic flexibility. Higher HRV generally indicates better vagal tone and regulatory capacity. While not all practices can implement HRV monitoring, even simple smartphone apps can provide useful baseline and progress data. Clients often find it validating to see objective evidence of their nervous system changes.

Self-report measures specific to autonomic states can complement traditional assessments. The Body Perception Questionnaire captures awareness of autonomic responses. The Polyvagal-informed assessments developed by Dana track state recognition and regulation capacity. These tools help clients become collaborators in tracking their progress.

Functional improvements often precede symptom reduction. A client might still have panic attacks but recover faster. They might still dissociate but recognize it happening and use resources to return. They might still get triggered but need less time to regulate. These incremental changes are crucial progress markers that traditional symptom measures might miss.

I track what I call "regulation resilience"—how quickly someone returns to baseline after activation. Initially, a trigger might dysregulate someone for days. With treatment, maybe it's hours, then minutes. This trajectory of faster recovery often predicts overall improvement and helps maintain hope during difficult periods.

Self-Care and Therapist Resilience

Working with trauma and dysregulated nervous systems affects our own autonomic state. According to research by Pearlman and Saakvitne on vicarious trauma, therapists' nervous systems can become dysregulated through repeated exposure to clients' traumatic material. But through a Polyvagal lens, we understand this isn't just psychological—it's biological resonance with dysregulated states.

Therapist self-care needs to address nervous system regulation specifically. It's not enough to think positively or take vacations if our nervous system is chronically activated. We need practices that directly support autonomic regulation: movement that discharges sympathetic activation, breathing practices that enhance vagal tone, relationships that provide co-regulation.

I structure my days with nervous system health in mind. Between difficult sessions, I do two minutes of breathing or movement. After particularly activating sessions, I might need vigorous walking to discharge energy. After sessions with dissociated clients, I might need energizing music to counter the pull toward shutdown. This isn't indulgence—it's maintaining my instrument.

According to research by Geller and Porges on therapeutic presence, our own regulation directly impacts our clinical effectiveness. We can't offer co-regulation from a dysregulated state. This makes our nervous system health an ethical imperative, not just personal wellness. Our regulated presence is often the most powerful intervention we provide.

Supervision and consultation through a Polyvagal lens focus on the therapist's autonomic responses. What triggers your sympathetic activation? Which clients pull you toward shutdown? How do you recognize your own state shifts? This somatic supervision helps therapists develop awareness of their patterns and resources for regulation.

Continuing Education and Resources

The field of Polyvagal-informed therapy is rapidly growing, with new research and applications emerging constantly. According to research by Porges and Dana on clinical applications, effective practice requires ongoing learning as our understanding of the nervous system expands.

Essential training includes not just theory but embodied practice. Reading about Polyvagal Theory provides intellectual understanding, but workshops that include experiential exercises develop the felt sense necessary for clinical application. Look for trainings that include practice time, not just lecture.

Integration with your existing modality matters. A CBT therapist might focus on how thoughts trigger state changes. A psychodynamic therapist might explore how early relationships shaped autonomic patterns. An EMDR therapist might track states during bilateral stimulation. The theory enhances what you already do rather than replacing it.

Professional communities provide crucial support. Online forums, consultation groups, and professional organizations offer spaces to discuss cases, share resources, and continue learning. The isolation of private practice can be particularly dysregulating, making professional connection essential for nervous system health.

Staying current with research is important but can be overwhelming. Following key researchers like Porges, Dana, and van der Kolk provides core updates. Journals like the International Journal of Psychophysiology and Clinical Social Work Journal regularly publish relevant research. But remember—not every study needs immediate integration into practice. Let the research settle, see what's replicated, focus on what's clinically relevant.

Creating Sustainable Practice

Building a Polyvagal-informed practice is an ongoing journey, not a destination. Each client teaches us something new about how nervous systems adapt and heal. Each session provides opportunities to refine our attunement and expand our skills. The learning never stops because nervous systems are endlessly complex and remarkably individual.

This approach requires holding multiple perspectives simultaneously—the psychological and the biological, the cognitive and the somatic, the individual and the relational. It asks us to be scientists observing autonomic states and artists creatively responding to what emerges. It demands both precision in tracking states and flexibility in intervention.

Most importantly, Polyvagal-informed practice asks us to trust the wisdom of the nervous system—both our clients' and our own. Symptoms that seemed like pathology reveal themselves as

163

protective adaptations. Resistance shows itself as nervous system wisdom. What looked like being stuck was actually the system protecting against overwhelm.

As you build your practice, be patient with yourself. You're not just learning new techniques—you're developing new ways of perceiving and responding. Your own nervous system needs time to integrate this approach. Start small, perhaps tracking states with one client before expanding. Notice what changes when you bring this awareness to your work.

The gift of Polyvagal-informed practice is that it makes us more human, not more technical. We're working with the same biological systems that govern our own regulation. We're all navigating the same challenges of staying regulated in a dysregulating world. This shared humanity, grounded in biological understanding, creates a foundation for healing that transcends any specific technique or intervention.

Chapter 21: Case Studies and Clinical Applications

Maria sat in my office for the fourth time, and something was different. For three sessions, she'd been locked in what I now recognized as chronic dorsal vagal shutdown—flat voice, minimal eye contact, describing years of childhood trauma as if reading a grocery list. But today, as she talked about her daughter's school play, I saw a flicker—her eyes brightened, her voice had a hint of melody, she actually smiled. For thirty seconds, she'd found ventral vagal. It was brief, but it was everything. It showed her nervous system still knew how to get there. We just had to help it remember the way.

Case studies bring theory to life, showing how Polyvagal principles translate into real clinical moments. Each client teaches us something new about how nervous systems adapt to trauma and find their way back to regulation. These aren't success stories where everything resolves neatly—they're real journeys with setbacks, surprises, and gradual transformation. Through these cases, we see how different presentations require different approaches, all guided by understanding the autonomic state beneath the symptoms.

What makes these cases powerful is seeing how Polyvagal awareness changes everything—assessment, intervention, even how we understand progress. A client who seems "resistant" reveals themselves as protecting against overwhelm. Someone who appears "unmotivated" shows themselves as stuck in shutdown. Symptoms that seemed random start making perfect sense when viewed through the lens of autonomic states.

Complex PTSD: Integrated Treatment Approach

James, a 45-year-old military veteran, came to therapy after his third divorce. "I destroy everything I touch," he said in our first session, his body rigid with tension. Traditional PTSD treatment had helped with nightmares but hadn't touched what he called "the ice inside." Through a Polyvagal lens, I saw someone oscillating between sympathetic hypervigilance and dorsal emotional shutdown, never finding the ventral vagal state where connection was possible.

According to research by Cloitre and colleagues on complex PTSD treatment, phase-based approaches that address nervous system regulation before trauma processing show better outcomes. With James, we needed to build basic regulation before touching trauma memories. His nervous system was like a smoke alarm that never stopped shrieking—we couldn't do repairs until we got the alarm to quiet down.

Phase one focused entirely on expanding his window of tolerance. We started with psychoeducation about his nervous system. When he understood that his "ice" was dorsal shutdown protecting him from overwhelming feelings, shame began to lift. He wasn't broken—his nervous system was doing exactly what it evolved to do. We mapped his triggers and glimmers, discovering that working on motorcycles was one of the few things that brought him into ventral vagal.

We used motorcycle maintenance as a metaphor and practice. The focused attention, the rhythm of mechanical work, the satisfaction of fixing something—all of this regulated his nervous system. We'd start sessions talking about his current project, letting his nervous system settle before approaching difficult material. This wasn't avoidance—it was building a ventral vagal platform from which he could eventually process trauma.

Phase two introduced somatic resourcing. James learned to recognize state shifts in his body. Tension in his jaw meant sympathetic activation building. Numbness in his chest signaled dorsal shutdown approaching. We developed state-specific interventions: cold water for rising activation, gentle movement for approaching shutdown, breathing practices for maintaining regulation.

Only after six months did we begin trauma processing, using a combination of EMDR and somatic experiencing. But now he had resources. When processing triggered sympathetic flooding, he could use his tools to regulate. When it triggered shutdown, he knew how to mobilize gently. The trauma didn't disappear, but his nervous system learned it could touch those memories without losing regulation completely.

Anxiety Disorders Through a Polyvagal Lens

Sarah, 28, had been diagnosed with generalized anxiety disorder, panic disorder, and social anxiety. Medication helped but didn't resolve the constant worry. Through a Polyvagal lens, I saw someone stuck in chronic sympathetic activation with periodic spikes into panic. Her nervous system had lost the ability to downregulate, like a car stuck in high gear.

According to research by Friedman on neurobiology of anxiety disorders, anxiety often involves compromised vagal brake function—the inability to inhibit sympathetic activation. Sarah's vagus nerve wasn't adequately suppressing her fight-or-flight response, leaving her in constant mobilization. Traditional anxiety treatment focused on thoughts, but we needed to work with her biology.

We started with HRV biofeedback, giving Sarah real-time data about her autonomic state. She could see how different breathing patterns immediately affected her nervous system. This wasn't just

167

relaxation—it was retraining her vagal brake. Within weeks, she could consciously shift her HRV, proving to her nervous system that regulation was possible.

Social situations were particularly triggering because her social engagement system was offline. Eye contact felt threatening, voices seemed too loud, friendly faces looked angry. We worked with this systematically. First, looking at photos of faces while regulated. Then videos without sound. Then videos with sound. Then real interactions in controlled doses. Each step taught her nervous system that social cues weren't dangerous.

The breakthrough came when she realized her anxiety had a protective function. Her sympathetic activation was trying to keep her safe from judgment and rejection—threats her nervous system remembered from childhood bullying. Once she understood this, she could appreciate her anxiety rather than fighting it. "Thank you for trying to protect me," she'd tell her activated state, "but I'm safe now."

Depression and Dorsal Vagal Dominance

Robert, 52, had been diagnosed with treatment-resistant depression. Fifteen years of various antidepressants, multiple therapists, even ECT hadn't helped. When I met him, he moved like he was underwater, spoke in monotone, and described feeling "dead inside but still walking around." Through a Polyvagal lens, this wasn't classic depression—it was chronic dorsal vagal shutdown.

According to research by Kolacz and colleagues on Polyvagal Theory and depression, what we call depression often involves dorsal vagal dominance—the nervous system stuck in conservation mode. Antidepressants might lift mood somewhat, but if the nervous system remains in shutdown, the person still feels disconnected and lifeless.

168

Traditional therapy had focused on his thoughts and behaviors, but Robert's thinking brain was barely online. In dorsal shutdown, the prefrontal cortex has minimal activity. Asking him to challenge negative thoughts was like asking someone in a coma to solve math problems. We needed to gently mobilize his nervous system first.

We started with tiny activations. Could he feel temperature differences? Could he notice the weight of his body in the chair? Each sensation, however small, was a victory—proof his nervous system could come online. We used music with strong rhythm to provide external activation his internal system couldn't generate.

Movement was crucial but had to be carefully titrated. Too much, and he'd collapse further. Too little, and nothing shifted. We started with seated movement—rolling shoulders, turning head, pressing feet into floor. Gradually building to standing, walking, eventually swimming. Each movement was teaching his nervous system that mobilization was safe.

The shift was gradual but profound. Color literally returned to his world—he started noticing beauty again. His voice developed inflection. He began feeling emotions—first irritation, then sadness, eventually even joy. The "depression" hadn't been a mood disorder but a nervous system stuck in shutdown. Once his nervous system learned to mobilize, his mood naturally improved.

Addiction Recovery and Nervous System Regulation

Lisa, 35, had been sober from alcohol for two years but was struggling. "I'm white-knuckling it every day," she said. "The only time I feel normal is when I'm running or in crisis at work." Through a Polyvagal lens, she was using external intensity to regulate internal chaos. Without alcohol to manage her nervous system, she'd found other ways to create the activation or numbing she needed.

According to research by Koob and Volkow on neurobiology of addiction, substance use often represents attempts to regulate dysregulated nervous systems. Alcohol might provide temporary ventral vagal mimicry—the relaxation and social ease that trauma survivors can't access naturally. Stimulants might lift people from dorsal shutdown. The substance isn't the problem—it's the solution to a nervous system problem.

Lisa's history revealed severe developmental trauma. Her nervous system had never learned to regulate naturally, so she'd found chemical regulation. Now sober, she was oscillating between sympathetic overdrive and dorsal collapse with no middle ground. The running and crisis-seeking were attempts to manage these swings.

We focused on building internal regulation rather than relying on external sources. This meant developing tolerance for ordinary states—not high, not low, just present. For someone whose nervous system knew only extremes, the middle felt intolerable at first. "It's so boring," she'd say about calm states. But boring was actually her nervous system learning a new possibility.

We used DBT skills through a Polyvagal lens. TIPP wasn't just distress tolerance—it was nervous system hacking. Mindfulness wasn't just awareness—it was ventral vagal cultivation. Interpersonal effectiveness wasn't just communication—it was social engagement system rehabilitation.

The key was helping Lisa understand that her addiction wasn't moral failure but nervous system adaptation. Her relapses weren't weakness but her system seeking regulation the only way it knew. This reframe dissolved shame and allowed her to approach recovery as nervous system healing rather than willpower battle.

Chronic Pain and Somatic Interventions

Michael, 40, had chronic back pain for ten years following a work injury. Multiple surgeries, physical therapy, and pain medication provided minimal relief. He was told it was "all in his head" when scans showed successful healing. Through a Polyvagal lens, the pain was real—his nervous system was stuck in a protective pattern that included pain as a danger signal.

According to research by Lumley and colleagues on emotional awareness and chronic pain, pain often involves not just tissue damage but nervous system sensitization. The nervous system becomes hypervigilant to bodily sensations, interpreting normal signals as dangerous. This isn't psychological—it's neurological protection gone haywire.

Michael's nervous system was in constant sympathetic activation, braced against pain that might come. This bracing created muscle tension that created more pain, creating a vicious cycle. Traditional pain management focused on reducing pain, but we needed to address the nervous system state maintaining it.

We started with somatic experiencing principles—tracking sensation without judgment. Instead of "pain," could he notice specific qualities? Sharp or dull? Moving or still? Hot or cold? This differentiation helped his nervous system stop lumping all sensation into the "danger" category.

Pendulation was crucial—moving attention between the pain area and neutral areas. This taught his nervous system that not everything hurt, that there were resources in his body. We'd spend time feeling his pain-free hand, his comfortable foot, building islands of safety in his body.

Movement exploration helped distinguish between protective bracing and actual limitation. When he moved slowly with awareness, he discovered more range than when he moved defensively. His nervous system was limiting movement to prevent anticipated pain, not because of actual tissue restriction.

Integration and Hope

These cases show that Polyvagal-informed treatment isn't a one-size-fits-all protocol but a flexible framework that adapts to each person's unique nervous system patterns. What they share is attention to autonomic states, respect for nervous system wisdom, and patience with the pace of biological change.

Each case also demonstrates that healing happens in relationship. The therapeutic relationship provides co-regulation that helps clients' nervous systems remember safety. But healing extends beyond therapy—to relationships, communities, and daily practices that support regulation.

Progress rarely follows a straight line. There are setbacks when life stressors narrow the window of tolerance. There are plateaus when the nervous system needs time to integrate changes. There are surprises when sudden shifts happen after months of apparent stasis. Understanding the biology helps us trust the process even when progress seems slow.

Most importantly, these cases show that change is possible even after decades of suffering. Nervous systems shaped by trauma can develop new patterns. Windows of tolerance can expand. People who've never felt safe can learn regulation. The capacity for healing is built into our biology—we just need to create the conditions for it to emerge.

As you work with your own clients, remember that each nervous system tells a unique story of adaptation and survival. Our job isn't to fix what's broken but to support the inherent healing capacity that never goes away. With patience, attunement, and understanding of the biology beneath the symptoms, transformation becomes possible.

Appendix A: Clinical Tools and Worksheets

Nervous System Mapping Templates

Personal Autonomic Map

Ventral Vagal (Safe and Social)

- Physical sensations when here:

- Thoughts that are possible:

- Emotions accessible:

- Behaviors exhibited:

- What brings me here:

- How long I can stay:

Sympathetic (Fight/Flight)

- Physical sensations when here:

- Thoughts that dominate:

- Emotions experienced:

- Behaviors exhibited:

- What triggers this state:

- What helps me down-regulate:

Dorsal Vagal (Shutdown)

- Physical sensations when here:

- Thoughts (or absence of):

- Emotions (or numbness):

- Behaviors exhibited:

- What triggers this state:

- What helps gentle mobilization:

Window of Tolerance Worksheets

Daily Window Tracker

- Morning width (1-10):

- Afternoon width (1-10):

- Evening width (1-10):

- What narrowed it today:

- What widened it today:

- State shifts noticed:

- Recovery times:

Co-Regulation Exercises

Partner Breathing

1. Sit facing each other

2. Place hands on own chest

3. Begin breathing audibly

4. Allow rhythms to naturally synchronize

5. Continue for 5 minutes

6. Share observations

State-Specific Intervention Guides

For Sympathetic Activation:

- Cold water on face/wrists
- Vigorous movement for 60 seconds
- Extended exhale breathing (4 in, 8 out)
- Bilateral stimulation (butterfly hug)
- Grounding (5-4-3-2-1 sensory)

For Dorsal Shutdown:

- Temperature change (warm/cool)
- Gentle movement (stretch, sway)
- Rhythmic stimulation (music, drumming)
- Sensory awakening (scents, textures)
- Orienting to environment

Client Psychoeducation Handouts

Understanding Your Nervous System States

Your nervous system has three main states, like gears in a car:

1. **Safe and Social** - You feel calm, connected, able to think clearly
2. **Fight or Flight** - You feel anxious, angry, need to move or act
3. **Shutdown** - You feel numb, disconnected, exhausted

These states aren't good or bad—they're your body's ways of protecting you.

Appendix B: Quick Reference Guides

Autonomic State Indicators

Visual Cues:

- Ventral: soft eyes, mobile face, relaxed posture

- Sympathetic: darting eyes, tense jaw, forward lean

- Dorsal: vacant stare, slack face, collapsed posture

Auditory Cues:

- Ventral: melodic voice, varied pace, clear articulation

- Sympathetic: rapid speech, elevated pitch, pressured quality

- Dorsal: monotone, slow/halting, weak volume

Intervention Selection Flowcharts

Client Presenting State?

├── Sympathetic Activation

│   ├── Discharge needed? → Movement/shaking

│   ├── Grounding needed? → 5-4-3-2-1 sensory

│   └── Soothing needed? → Extended exhale/cold water

├── Dorsal Shutdown

│   ├── Gentle activation? → Temperature/rhythm

│   ├── Orientation needed? → Environmental awareness

│   └── Movement possible? → Slow stretching

└── Mixed State

    ├── Identify dominant → Target that first

    └── Stabilize before processing

Crisis Intervention Strategies

Immediate Stabilization:

1. Ensure physical safety

2. Use calm, steady voice

3. Minimize stimulation

4. Offer co-regulation through presence

5. Simple orienting (name, place, date)

6. Basic breathing together

7. No processing until regulated

Telehealth Adaptations

Creating Safety Through Screens:

- Stable internet (reduce disconnection anxiety)

- Consistent background (predictable environment)

- Good lighting on face (social engagement cues visible)

- Clear audio (prosody transmitted)

- Regular check-ins about connection quality

- Backup plan if technology fails

Appendix C: Resources and Training

Professional Organizations and Certification Programs

- Polyvagal Institute (Stephen Porges and Deb Dana)

- Somatic Experiencing International

- Sensorimotor Psychotherapy Institute

- International Association of Trauma Professionals

- EMDR International Association

Recommended Readings and Research

Foundational Texts:

- Porges, S. (2011). The Polyvagal Theory

- Dana, D. (2018). The Polyvagal Theory in Therapy

- van der Kolk, B. (2014). The Body Keeps the Score

- Levine, P. (2010). In an Unspoken Voice

- Ogden, P. (2015). Sensorimotor Psychotherapy

Online Resources and Communities

- Polyvagal Institute website and resources

- Trauma Research Foundation

- National Center for PTSD

- International Society for Traumatic Stress Studies

- Clinical online forums and consultation groups

Training Opportunities in Integrated Approaches

Core Trainings:

- Polyvagal Theory basics (2-day workshops)
- Clinical applications (multi-day intensives)
- Somatic approaches integration
- Trauma-informed yoga certification
- EMDR with Polyvagal integration

Supervision and Consultation Resources

Finding Polyvagal-Informed Supervision:

- Check Polyvagal Institute directory
- Regional trauma-informed supervisor lists
- Online consultation groups
- Peer consultation circles
- Mentorship programs through training institutes

References

- Beauchaine, T. P., & Thayer, J. F. (2015). Heart rate variability as a transdiagnostic biomarker of psychopathology. *International Journal of Psychophysiology, 98*(2, Pt 2), 338–350.

- Bellato, A., Arora, I., Hollis, C., & Groom, M. J. (2020). Is autonomic nervous system function atypical in attention deficit hyperactivity disorder (ADHD)? A systematic review of the evidence. *Neuroscience & Biobehavioral Reviews, 108*, 182–206.

- Berntson, G. G., & Cacioppo, J. T. (2004). Heart rate variability: Stress and psychiatric conditions. In M. Malik & A. J. Camm (Eds.), *Dynamic electrocardiography* (pp. 57–64). Blackwell.

- Blaustein, M. E., & Kinniburgh, K. M. (2018). *Treating traumatic stress in children and adolescents: How to foster resilience through attachment, self-regulation, and competency* (2nd ed.). Guilford Press.

- Bremner, J. D. (2006). Traumatic stress: Effects on the brain. *Dialogues in Clinical Neuroscience, 8*(4), 445–461.

- Brom, D., Stokar, Y., Lawi, C., Nuriel-Porat, V., Ziv, Y., Lerner, K., & Ross, G. (2017). Somatic Experiencing for posttraumatic stress disorder: A randomized controlled outcome study. *Journal of Traumatic Stress, 30*(3), 304–312.

- Brown, K. W., & Ryan, R. M. (2003). The benefits of being present: Mindfulness and its role in psychological well-being. *Journal of Personality and Social Psychology, 84*(4), 822–848.

- Brown, R. P., & Gerbarg, P. L. (2005). Sudarshan Kriya yogic breathing in the treatment of stress, anxiety, and depression: Part I—Neurophysiologic model. *Journal of Alternative and Complementary Medicine, 11*(1), 189–201.

- Cloitre, M., Courtois, C. A., Ford, J. D., Green, B. L., Alexander, P., Briere, J., ... Van der Hart, O. (2012). *The ISTSS expert consensus treatment guidelines for complex PTSD in adults.* International Society for Traumatic Stress Studies.

- Cook, A., Spinazzola, J., Ford, J., Lanktree, C., Blaustein, M., Cloitre, M., ... van der Kolk, B. (2005). Complex trauma in children and adolescents. *Psychiatric Annals, 35*(5), 390–398.

- Corrigan, F. M., Fisher, J. J., & Nutt, D. J. (2011). Autonomic dysregulation and the window of tolerance model of the effects of complex emotional trauma. *Journal of Psychopharmacology, 25*(1), 17–25.

- Cozolino, L. (2014). *The neuroscience of human relationships: Attachment and the developing social brain* (2nd ed.). W. W. Norton & Company.

- Craig, A. D. (2009). How do you feel—now? The anterior insula and human awareness. *Nature Reviews Neuroscience, 10*(1), 59–70.

- Dana, D. (2018). *The polyvagal theory in therapy: Engaging the rhythm of regulation.* W. W. Norton & Company.

- Dana, D. (2020). *Polyvagal exercises for safety and connection: 50 client-centered practices*. W. W. Norton & Company.

- Dale, L. P., Carroll, L. E., Galen, G., Hayes, J. A., Webb, K. W., & Porges, S. W. (2009). Abuse history is related to autonomic regulation to mild exercise and psychological well-being. *Applied Psychophysiology and Biofeedback, 34*(4), 299–308.

- Emerson, D., & Hopper, E. (2011). *Overcoming trauma through yoga: Reclaiming your body*. North Atlantic Books.

- Feldman, R. (2012). Parent-infant synchrony: A biobehavioral model of mutual influences in the formation of affiliative bonds. *Monographs of the Society for Research in Child Development, 77*(2), 42–51.

- Field, T. (2010). Touch for socioemotional and physical well-being: A review. *Developmental Review, 30*(4), 367–382.

- Fisher, J. (2017). *Healing the fragmented selves of trauma survivors: Overcoming internal self-alienation*. Routledge.

- Flores, P. J., & Porges, S. W. (2017). Group psychotherapy as a neural exercise: Bridging polyvagal theory and attachment theory. *International Journal of Group Psychotherapy, 67*(2), 202–222.

- Fonseca, A., Osma, J., Moreno-Peral, P., & Barrera, A. Z. (2021). Dance/movement therapy for improving psychological and physical outcomes in cancer patients: A systematic review and meta-analysis. *International Journal of Environmental Research and Public Health, 18*(20), 10742.

- Fosha, D. (2000). *The transforming power of affect: A model for accelerated change*. Basic Books.

- Friedman, B. H. (2007). An autonomic flexibility–neurovisceral integration model of anxiety and cardiac vagal tone. *Biological Psychology, 74*(2), 185–199.

- Gallese, V. (2009). Mirror neurons, embodied simulation, and the neural basis of social identification. *Psychoanalytic Dialogues, 19*(5), 519–536.

- Geller, S. M., & Porges, S. W. (2014). Therapeutic presence: Neurophysiological mechanisms mediating feeling safe in therapeutic relationships. *Journal of Psychotherapy Integration, 24*(3), 178–192).

- Gendlin, E. T. (1996). *Focusing-oriented psychotherapy: A manual of the experiential method*. Guilford Press.

- Gerritsen, R. J. S., & Band, G. P. H. (2018). Breath of life: The respiratory vagal stimulation model of contemplative activity. *Frontiers in Human Neuroscience, 12*, 397.

- Gilbert, P. (2009). *The compassionate mind: A new approach to life's challenges*. Constable & Robinson.

- Hanna, T. (1990). Clinical somatic education: A new discipline in the field of health care. *Somatics: Magazine-Journal of the Bodily Arts and Sciences, 8*(1), 4–10.

- Hass-Cohen, N., & Carr, R. (Eds.). (2008). *Art therapy and clinical neuroscience*. Jessica Kingsley Publishers.

- Hasson, U., Ghazanfar, A. A., Galantucci, B., Garrod, S., & Keysers, C. (2012). Brain-to-brain coupling: A mechanism for creating and sharing a social world. *Trends in Cognitive Sciences, 16*(2), 114–121.

- Heaphy, E. D., & Dutton, J. E. (2008). Positive social interactions and the human body at work: Linking organizations and physiology. *Academy of Management Review, 33*(1), 137–162.

- Hobfoll, S. E., Watson, P., Bell, C. C., Bryant, R. A., Brymer, M. J., Friedman, M. J., … Ursano, R. J. (2007). Five essential elements of immediate and mid-term mass trauma intervention: Empirical evidence. *Psychiatry, 70*(4), 283–315.

- Hofmann, S. G., & Otto, M. W. (2008). *Cognitive behavioral therapy for social anxiety disorder: Evidence-based and disorder-specific treatment techniques*. Routledge.

- Jarero, I., & Artigas, L. (2010). The EMDR integrative group treatment protocol: Application with adults during ongoing geopolitical crisis. *Journal of EMDR Practice and Research, 4*(4), 148–155.

- Kabat-Zinn, J. (2003). Mindfulness-based interventions in context: Past, present, and future. *Clinical Psychology: Science and Practice, 10*(2), 144–156.

- Kearney, D. J., McManus, C., Malte, C. A., Martinez, M. E., Felleman, B., & Simpson, T. L. (2014). Loving-kindness meditation and the broaden-and-build theory of positive emotions among veterans with posttraumatic stress disorder. *Medical Care, 52*(12, Suppl. 5), S32–S38.

- Kemp, A. H., & Quintana, D. S. (2013). The relationship between mental and physical health: Insights from the study of heart rate variability. *International Journal of Psychophysiology, 89*(3), 288–296.

- Kolacz, J., Kovacic, K. K., & Porges, S. W. (2019). Traumatic stress and the autonomic brain–gut connection in development: Polyvagal theory as an integrative framework for psychosocial and gastrointestinal pathology. *Developmental Psychobiology, 61*(5), 796–809.

- Kok, B. E., & Fredrickson, B. L. (2010). Upward spirals of the heart: Autonomic flexibility, as indexed by vagal tone, reciprocally and prospectively predicts positive emotions and social connectedness. *Biological Psychology, 85*(3), 432–436.

- Koob, G. F., & Volkow, N. D. (2016). Neurobiology of addiction: A neurocircuitry analysis. *The Lancet Psychiatry, 3*(8), 760–773.

- Korn, D. L., & Leeds, A. M. (2002). Preliminary evidence of efficacy for EMDR resource development and installation in the stabilization phase of treatment of complex posttraumatic stress disorder. *Journal of Clinical Psychology, 58*(12), 1465–1487.

- Kozlowska, K., Walker, P., McLean, L., & Carrive, P. (2015). Fear and the defense cascade: Clinical implications and management. *Harvard Review of Psychiatry, 23*(4), 263–287.

- Kreibig, S. D. (2010). Autonomic nervous system activity in emotion: A review. *Biological Psychology, 84*(3), 394–421.

- Kuhfuß, M., Maldei, T., Hetmanek, A., & Baumann, N. (2021). Somatic Experiencing—Effectiveness and key factors of a body-oriented trauma therapy: A scoping literature review. *European Journal of Psychotraumatology, 12*(1), 1929023.

- Laborde, S., Mosley, E., & Thayer, J. F. (2017). Heart rate variability and cardiac vagal tone in psychophysiological research—Recommendations for experiment planning, data analysis, and data reporting. *Frontiers in Psychology, 8*, 213.

- Lanius, R. A., Bluhm, R., & Frewen, P. A. (2011). How understanding the neurobiology of complex post-traumatic stress disorder can inform clinical practice: A social cognitive and affective neuroscience approach. *Acta Psychiatrica Scandinavica, 124*(5), 331–348.

- Lanius, R. A., Vermetten, E., Loewenstein, R. J., Brand, B., Schmahl, C., Bremner, J. D., & Spiegel, D. (2010). Emotion modulation in PTSD: Clinical and neurobiological evidence for a dissociative subtype. *American Journal of Psychiatry, 167*(6), 640–647).

- Levine, P. A. (1997). *Waking the tiger: Healing trauma.* North Atlantic Books.

- Levine, P. A. (2010). *In an unspoken voice: How the body releases trauma and restores goodness.* North Atlantic Books.

- Linehan, M. M. (1993). *Cognitive-behavioral treatment of borderline personality disorder.* Guilford Press.

- Lumley, M. A., Cohen, J. L., Borszcz, G. S., Cano, A., Radcliffe, A. M., Porter, L. S., … Keefe, F. J. (2011). Pain and emotion: A biopsychosocial review of recent research. *Journal of Clinical Psychology, 67*(9), 942–968.

- Lunkenheimer, E., Kemp, C. J., Lucas-Thompson, R. G., Cole, P. M., & Albrecht, E. C. (2017). Assessing biobehavioral self-regulation and coregulation in early childhood: The Parent–Child Challenge Task. *Infant and Child Development, 26*(1), e1965.

- Maté, G. (2003). *When the body says no: The cost of hidden stress.* Knopf Canada.

- McCraty, R., & Shaffer, F. (2015). Heart rate variability: New perspectives on physiological mechanisms, assessment of self-regulatory capacity, and health risk. *Global Advances in Health and Medicine, 4*(1), 46–61.

- Mehling, W. E., Price, C., Daubenmier, J. J., Acree, M., Bartmess, E., & Stewart, A. (2012). The Multidimensional Assessment of Interoceptive Awareness (MAIA). *PLoS ONE, 7*(11), e48230.

- Menakem, R. (2017). *My grandmother's hands: Racialized trauma and the pathway to mending our hearts and bodies.* Central Recovery Press.

- Najavits, L. M. (2002). *Seeking safety: A treatment manual for PTSD and substance abuse.* Guilford Press.

- Neff, K. D. (2003). Self-compassion: An alternative conceptualization of a healthy attitude toward oneself. *Self and Identity, 2*(2), 85–101.

- Nijenhuis, E. R., Vanderlinden, J., & Spinhoven, P. (1998). Animal defensive reactions as a model for trauma-induced dissociative reactions. *Journal of Traumatic Stress, 11*(2), 243–260.

- Ogden, P., Minton, K., & Pain, C. (2006). *Trauma and the body: A sensorimotor approach to psychotherapy.* W. W. Norton & Company.

- Ogden, P., & Fisher, J. (2015). *Sensorimotor psychotherapy: Interventions for trauma and attachment.* W. W. Norton & Company.

- Payne, P., Levine, P. A., & Crane-Godreau, M. A. (2015). Somatic Experiencing: Using interoception and proprioception as core elements of trauma therapy. *Frontiers in Psychology, 6*, 93.

- Pearlman, L. A., & Saakvitne, K. W. (1995). *Trauma and the therapist: Countertransference and vicarious traumatization in psychotherapy with incest survivors.* W. W. Norton & Company.

- Perry, B. D., & Szalavitz, M. (2006). *The boy who was raised as a dog: And other stories from a child psychiatrist's notebook.* Basic Books.

- Pinderhughes, H., Davis, R., & Williams, M. (2015). *Adverse community experiences and resilience: A framework for addressing and preventing community trauma.* Prevention Institute.

- Porges, S. W. (1995). Orienting in a defensive world: Mammalian modifications of our evolutionary heritage—A polyvagal theory. *Psychophysiology, 32*(4), 301–318.

- Porges, S. W. (2001). The polyvagal theory: Phylogenetic substrates of a social nervous system. *International Journal of Psychophysiology, 42*(2), 123–146.

- Porges, S. W. (2003). Social engagement and attachment: A phylogenetic perspective. *Annals of the New York Academy of Sciences, 1008*(1), 31–47.

- Porges, S. W. (2004). Neuroception: A subconscious system for detecting threats and safety. *Zero to Three, 24*(5), 19–24.

- Porges, S. W. (2007). The polyvagal perspective. *Biological Psychology, 74*(2), 116–143.

- Porges, S. W. (2009). The polyvagal theory: New insights into adaptive reactions of the autonomic nervous system.

Cleveland Clinic Journal of Medicine, 76(Suppl. 2), S86–S90.

- Porges, S. W. (2011). *The polyvagal theory: Neurophysiological foundations of emotions, attachment, communication, and self-regulation.* W. W. Norton & Company.

- Porges, S. W. (2022). Polyvagal theory: A science of safety. *Frontiers in Integrative Neuroscience, 16*, 871227.

- Porges, S. W., Bazhenova, O. V., Bal, E., Carlson, N., Sorokin, Y., Heilman, K. J., Cook, E. H., & Lewis, G. F. (2014). Reducing auditory hypersensitivities in autistic spectrum disorder: Preliminary findings evaluating the Listening Project Protocol. *Frontiers in Pediatrics, 2*, 80.

- Porges, S. W., & Buczynski, R. (2012). *The polyvagal theory for treating trauma: A teleseminar session.* National Institute for the Clinical Application of Behavioral Medicine. [Transcript/grey literature]

- Porges, S. W., & Lewis, G. F. (2010). The polyvagal hypothesis: Common mechanisms mediating autonomic regulation, vocalizations, and listening. In *Handbook of Behavioral Neuroscience* (Vol. 19, pp. 255–264).

- Rhodes, A. M., Spinazzola, J., van der Kolk, B. A., et al. (2016). Yoga for adult women with chronic PTSD: Long-term follow-up of a randomized controlled trial. *Journal of Alternative and Complementary Medicine, 22*(3), 189–196. *(Optional companion to 2014 RCT)*

- Rothschild, B. (2000). *The body remembers: The psychophysiology of trauma and trauma treatment.* W. W. Norton & Company.

- Safer, D. L., Adler, S., & Masson, P. C. (2018). *The DBT solution for emotional eating: A proven program to break the cycle of bingeing and out-of-control eating.* Guilford Press.

- Sander, E. J., Caza, A., & Jordan, P. J. (2019). Psychological perceptions matter: Developing the reactions to the physical work environment scale. *Building and Environment, 148,* 338–347.

- Scaer, R. (2014). *The body bears the burden: Trauma, dissociation, and disease* (3rd ed.). Routledge.

- Schore, A. N. (2001). Effects of a secure attachment relationship on right brain development, affect regulation, and infant mental health. *Infant Mental Health Journal, 22*(1–2), 7–66.

- Schore, A. N. (2003). *Affect dysregulation and disorders of the self.* W. W. Norton & Company.

- Schore, A. N. (2012). *The science of the art of psychotherapy.* W. W. Norton & Company.

- Schwartz, R. C. (1995). *Internal family systems therapy.* Guilford Press.

- Schwartz, R. C., & Sweezy, M. (2020). *Internal family systems therapy* (2nd ed.). Guilford Press.

- Shaffer, F., & Ginsberg, J. P. (2017). An overview of heart rate variability metrics and norms. *Frontiers in Public Health, 5,* 258.

- Shapiro, F. (2001). *Eye movement desensitization and reprocessing (EMDR): Basic principles, protocols, and procedures* (2nd ed.). Guilford Press.

- Siegel, D. J. (1999). *The developing mind: How relationships and the brain interact to shape who we are.* Guilford Press.

- Siegel, D. J. (2010). *Mindsight: The new science of personal transformation.* Bantam Books.

- Siegel, D. J. (2012). *The developing mind: How relationships and the brain interact to shape who we are* (2nd ed.). Guilford Press.

- Siegel, D. J., & Solomon, M. (Eds.). (2003). *Healing trauma: Attachment, mind, body, and brain.* W. W. Norton & Company.

- Sullivan, M. B., Erb, M., Schmalzl, L., Moonaz, S., Noggle Taylor, J., & Porges, S. W. (2018). Yoga therapy and polyvagal theory: The convergence of traditional wisdom and contemporary neuroscience for self-regulation and resilience. *Frontiers in Human Neuroscience, 12*, 67.

- Teicher, M. H., & Samson, J. A. (2016). Annual research review: Enduring neurobiological effects of childhood abuse and neglect. *Journal of Child Psychology and Psychiatry, 57*(3), 241–266.

- Tronick, E. (2007). *The neurobehavioral and social-emotional development of infants and children.* W. W. Norton & Company.

- Tronick, E., & Beeghly, M. (2011). Infants' meaning-making and the development of mental health problems. *American Psychologist, 66*(2), 107–119.

- van der Hart, O., Nijenhuis, E. R., & Steele, K. (2006). *The haunted self: Structural dissociation and the treatment of chronic traumatization.* W. W. Norton & Company.

- van de Kamp, M. M., Scheffers, M., Hatzmann, J., Emck, C., Cuijpers, P., & Beek, P. J. (2019). Body- and movement-oriented interventions for posttraumatic stress disorder: A systematic review and meta-analysis. Journal of Traumatic Stress, 32(6), 967–976.

- van de Kamp, M., Emck, C., Scheffers, M., Hoven, M., Cuijpers, P., & Beek, P. J. (2025). Psychomotor therapy for posttraumatic stress disorder. Body, Movement and Dance in Psychotherapy, 20(3), 231–249. (Epub Dec 6, 2024).

- van der Kolk, B. A. (2014). *The body keeps the score: Brain, mind, and body in the healing of trauma*. Viking.

- van der Kolk, B. A., & Fisler, R. (1995). Dissociation and the fragmentary nature of traumatic memories: Overview and exploratory study. *Journal of Traumatic Stress, 8*(4), 505–525.

- van der Kolk, B. A., Stone, L., West, J., Rhodes, A. M., Emerson, D., Suvak, M., & Spinazzola, J. (2014). Yoga as an adjunctive treatment for posttraumatic stress disorder: A randomized controlled trial. *Journal of Clinical Psychiatry, 75*(6), e559–e565.

- Vaschillo, E. G., Vaschillo, B., & Lehrer, P. M. (2006). Characteristics of resonance in heart rate variability stimulated by biofeedback. *Applied Psychophysiology and Biofeedback, 31*(2), 129–142.

- Wendt, D. C., Gone, J. P., & Nagata, D. K. (2015). Potentially harmful therapy and multicultural counseling: Bridging two disciplinary discourses. *The Counseling Psychologist, 43*(3), 334–358.

- Williamson, J. B., Heilman, K. M., Porges, E. C., Lamb, D. G., & Porges, S. W. (2013). A possible mechanism for PTSD symptoms in patients with traumatic brain injury: Central autonomic network disruption. *Frontiers in Neuroengineering, 6,* 13.

- Wylie, M. S., & Turner, L. (2011). The attuned therapist: Does attachment theory really matter? *Psychotherapy Networker, 35*(2), 19–27.

* 9 7 8 1 9 2 3 6 0 4 9 8 8 *